CIRCLE OF HOPE

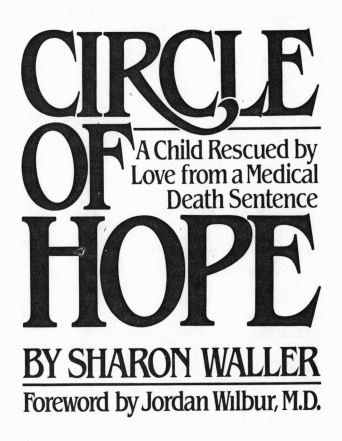

CIRCLE OF HOPE

A Child Rescued by
Love from a Medical
Death Sentence

BY SHARON WALLER

Foreword by Jordan Wilbur, M.D.

M. EVANS AND COMPANY, INC.
New York

Library of Congress Cataloging in Publication Data

Waller, Sharon.
  Circle of hope.

    1. Cancer—Patients—United States—Biography.
2. Bones—Cancer.   3. Halper, Jobi, 1963-
3. Osteosarcoma.   4. Tumors in children—United States—
Biography.   I. Title.
RC280.B6W34   362.1'9892994'00924   81-9846

ISBN 0-87131-355-3   AACR2

M. Evans and Company, Inc.
216 East 49 Street
New York, New York 10017

Design by Diane Gedymin

Manufactured in the United States of America

9 8 7 6 5 4 3 2 1

Author's Note

The names of all doctors, medical centers, and hospitals in Minneapolis have been changed. For their privacy, I have also changed the names of patients and doctors in Palo Alto. But Dr. Jordan Wilbur and all my friends and family are represented by their own names.

I DEDICATE THIS BOOK

to Heidi and Jonathan Halper, who sacrificed a piece of childhood . . .

to Helen Rosen, who suffered, loved, and grew . . .

to Dr. Jordan Wilbur, who believes in life . . .

to Joel Waller, who believes in me . . .

to Jobi, who shines

FOREWORD

THE DIAGNOSIS OF CANCER in anyone in your family creates a reaction of overwhelming fear and helplessness. This reaction is even more severe when it is your child that has the cancer. Sharon Waller has described vividly the emotional storm that engulfed her family as waves of helplessness and despair threatened to overcome them. The bonds of family love helped to hold them together, as they refused to accept the apparent inevitable outcome, and with courage and perserverance sought a way to overcome the disease that threatened the life of their child. This drama has occurred on many occasions as families seek to combine their love and support with the medical advances being achieved by scientists from all over the world, and to merge these great forces into a circle of people who can work together to provide real hope for the child whose life is threatened.

Medical progress has brought about a remarkable change in the results of treatment of children with cancer over the past ten years. What was usually regarded as a fatal disease can now be considered a life-threatening disease. A number of changes have occurred that now enable at least half of all children with cancer who are treated at a major children's cancer center, to be alive and well five years later, with a good chance to live a full lifetime. These factors include new drugs, progress in the knowledge of how to use the drugs more effectively, and better supportive care, such as better antibiotics, blood transfusions and intravenous feedings, to manage the complications of the cancers and the treatments.

Of greater importance has been a change in attitude and

philosophy on the part of the health care professionals. This includes treating all patients with the plan to eradicate their cancer and help them get well, regardless of the type, location, or extent of spread of the cancer. We know that we cannot successfully eradicate the disease in every patient, but we should try. It is only if we try that it is possible for it to happen. If the known treatment for a particular cancer is not usually effective, then if we are to have a real chance to eradicate the disease, we must try some new form of therapy that offers some possibility of a better response.

The change in results from the treatment of young people with osteosarcoma is an example of the progress that has occurred. About ten years ago, most physicians regarded osteosarcoma as a usually fatal disease, from which only a small percentage of patients were cured by radical surgery, usually amputation. Spread of disease to the lungs usually occurred within months and was rapidly fatal. Improved aggressive chemotherapy has now prevented this problem in many patients. More accurate diagnostic studies combined with skilled lung surgery and chemotherapy have helped save many others when the disease has spread to the lungs. Recently, in several treatment centers chemotherapy is being combined with "limb salvage surgery" to avoid amputation. With this technique, the patient is initially treated with chemotherapy. The residual area of tumor in the bone is then removed and usually replaced with a custom-made metal bone. With these advances, the vast majority of young people with osteosarcoma can now be successfully treated without requiring amputation.

In order to have the best chance for success we must enlist the help of everyone who has something to contribute. At the Children's Cancer Research Institute in San Francisco, this includes the patient and the patient's family. They are vital members of our health care team. No one has a greater interest in the outcome of the therapy or the side effects of the treatments than the patient and the patient's family. No one knows the patient better or can care for the child as well as the child's family. They have a lot to teach the health care team about what works best for the patient, and in turn the health care team members have a lot to teach the patient and the family. The doctors, nurses, and other health professionals should work hand in hand with the patient and the family to achieve their common goal of eradication of the child's disease. This goal includes the minimization of side effects and the return to a normal life-style as quickly as possible.

Here at our hospital, family members are encouraged to continue in their traditional role of caring for the child, and not to turn this responsibility over to the hospital staff. The hospital staff is encouraged to work with the patient and family, providing their medical skills and knowledge to help solve the problems. This means working *with* people, rather than doing things *to* them. When patients and family members have an opportunity to work hand in hand with the medical and nursing staff, they also learn about the disease, the treatment and their effects. This involvement allows them to give "informed consent" more readily when new and experimental treatments or tests are proposed as part of the child's care.

Sometimes it is not possible for parents to stay in the hospital with their child. Frequently a grandparent, older sibling, or another family member or close friend can stay and be the family advocate. It is often of value for a brother or sister to stay. This allows the sibling to be an important part of caring for the patient and helps maintain a more normal family atmosphere in the hospital. The families in the hospital are often able to provide strength, support and information not only for the members of their own family, but also for the other families who share similar burdens.

Just as the families provide support for each other, the medical staff also becomes involved in providing skills and support that are all directed toward a common goal. This goal is the ultimate physical and emotional recovery of the child, and of the family as well. Each year we achieve this goal more often, but we should not be satisfied until every child with cancer can be successfully treated. Working toward this goal, physicians, nurses and families should join with other health professionals to form a circle of hope and love around each child. With this kind of care and support every child with cancer has a better chance to do well. The story of Jobi Halper shows how it can happen.

JORDAN R. WILBUR, M.D.
Executive Director
Children's Cancer Research Institute
Pacific Medical Center
San Francisco

PART ONE

1

THE ONLY THING I didn't like about his office was the poster on the wall. I knew it was there to inspire, but it made me uncomfortable. There was a desperate-looking cat hanging from a ledge by its front claws. The caption read, "Hang in There Baby." Well, the cat didn't have much choice, did it? It was hang in there or fall. Fall to what? And maybe falling wasn't much worse than what it was costing that cat to hang on. As I said, I wished the poster hadn't been there.

But Dr. Jordan Wilbur I liked. He should have been on the wall inspiring confidence. God, he was big. About six two. Wide shoulders under that white lab coat; big, gentle hands. Was he forty? Maybe forty-five. It didn't matter. Old enough to be comforting, young enough to understand. He was handsome, in a strong crinkly-eyed, touch-of-gray sort of way.

It made me feel good when he said, "All the children here have a problem." Problem . . . get it? Right away you have something with a solution. Hey, children can't die of a problem, can they? Not the children. Not Jobi.

Jobi. She was outside the office somewhere looking at Shirley Temple's doll collection. On her crutches. It was wonderful of Ms. Temple to give her beautiful dolls to the Children's Hospital at Stanford. Everyone loved them. It gave visitors something to think about besides broken bones, asthma, and other, worse things.

There were many kinds of sick children at the hospital. But Dr. Wilbur was in charge of only one unit . . . a rather small one. It was the oncology floor. All his children had the same problem. They had cancer.

What was Jobi doing there? I asked God and myself that question a lot.

Jobi. She was really named Jo Beth, after my two favorite Little Women and David's grandmother. But mostly we called her Sunshine. I'm not sure when or why we started calling her that. Maybe because she had long silken hair all streaked with morning light. Her skin was peach, and even her blue eyes had flecks of honey. Or was it the smile? When Jobi smiled, her face opened like a flower and glowed with an inner light. She was a golden soul from the moment of her birth.

2

OUR RAY OF SUNSHINE was born by cesarean section on a bright April morning. She weighed six pounds and had yellow hair, blue eyes, and little flower lips. When I took her in my arms, she nestled under my chin and smelled like powder. Jobi.

When Jobi was two, she looked like Tinkerbell. A tiny person with shaggy, shimmery hair and round eyes. Even then, people gravitated toward her. There was a magic aura surrounding this child.

Sunshine. Her nursery school teacher called her that. One day I went to the school for a conference. Jobi's teacher and I watched her through a one-way mirror. We could see the class, but the children had no idea they were being observed.

Jobi pranced about the room, laughing her tinkly laugh. Other children followed her, laughing too. She threw her

4

arms in the air and twirled around. The others twirled with her. Then, with a squeal, she plopped to the ground, her dress floating up, her straight fine hair flying. All the children went tumbling down with her, amid little shrieks and laughs and jumbles of small arms and legs.

"She lights up the room." The teacher smiled.

The summer after Jobi's eighth birthday, in 1971, was a difficult one for David and me. Our marriage was troubled and we were not happy. David resented the time I devoted to writing and directing shows in the community, and I, in turn, chafed under his disapproval, longing for affection he seemed unable to give.

I recall trying to fill my life with beauty. I bought long airy dresses for my little girls, Heidi and Jobi, and left their blond hair loose to fly in the wind. I planted flowers everywhere I could and taught my four-year-old son, Jonathan, to pat earth over the roots. I wrote song lyrics and played the piano. But a cloud seemed to hover over us. David and I were on parallel lines and I couldn't touch him.

I still have a vision of Jobi that summer. She's barefoot— her toes just peeking from under a white dress of fine soft cotton so thin it floats. Her hair is streaked by the sun; it is pulled back from her round, golden forehead and hanging nearly to her hips. She twirls in my big round flower garden, dancing to music no one else can hear.

Fall came and life grew darker. One night I stood at the kitchen counter tearing lettuce for dinner. I looked up and saw Jobi standing there. She was staring at me and her face was a shadow.

"Something wrong?"

She shrugged and her eyes didn't meet mine. Strange reticence from the usual chatterbox. She continued to stand there.

"A boy kicked me today," she finally offered.

"Oh? That wasn't nice of him," I replied, wondering if I had enough potato flakes for dinner.

"In the knee," she said softly.

"Hmmm?" I rummaged in my chaotic cupboard for a can of peas. I had been working on a new musical for a country club group all afternoon, and dinner would be late and less than gourmet.

"He kicked me in the knee." She said this a little louder. I turned.

"Let me see."

The child solemnly pulled up the hem of her red, pleated skirt and thrust her still suntanned leg in front of me. There was no mark.

"I think you're gonna live." I smiled and pronounced the parental inanity.

She looked at me reproachfully and left the room.

The next morning I handed her a lunch sack. I felt groggy. David and I had quarreled far into the night because I neglected the house while I was writing or, as in this case, was directing a show. As usual, nothing was resolved and the morning found me still smarting from bitter remarks. Children are often infected with their parents' moods, and Heidi had left for school early, in a huff because I was out of the kind of jelly she liked in her sandwich. She wouldn't have waited for Jobi in any case. A sixth grader would never be seen in the company of a third grader.

I looked at my small son with exasperation. Jonathan was still wearing his pajamas and was eating his cereal one flake at a time. His nursery school bus was due in fifteen minutes. It was so like this cheerful, pleasant little boy to ignore pressure around him and concentrate on the pleasure life had to offer. Unlike his blond, blue-eyed sisters, one moody and introspective, the other frantically energetic, the son had emerged with dark brown hair, eyes like chocolate almonds, and a permanent easy-going smile on his face. I was about to prod him into action when Jobi interrupted me.

"My knee still hurts."

I smiled at her.

"That boy must have kicked you pretty hard. Well, it will probably take a few days till it feels better."

She didn't smile when she left that morning, but she was limping slightly. Engrossed in my problems, I dismissed the hurt knee from my mind.

A few days later Jobi came home from school and said, "I didn't go to gym today."

"Oh? Why not?" Jobi always loved gym. She was naturally agile and had great balance. When she was very small, David taught her to stand on his outstretched hands. He could walk around the house with her perched on his palms.

Jobi looked at me sadly. "My leg hurts too much to go to gym."

I wasn't overly concerned, but I decided to take her to see our doctor.

3

DR. JOSEPHINE PARRISH was an attractive woman of forty with short crisp brown hair and intelligent brown eyes behind wire-framed glasses. Her successful pediatric practice resulted from her kindly but firm handling of children and their mothers as well as complete medical competence. She carefully examined Jobi, including the offending knee.

"Do I get an operation?" Jobi asked fearfully.

"No." The understanding doctor smiled. "You get a kiss." She set Jobi on the ground and kissed her cheek. "Now you go tell the nurse I said you're to have two suckers today."

A small smile, and Jobi limped out of the room toward the nurse's station.

"What do you think?" I asked.

"The knee is fine. I don't see a thing."

"Then why the limp?"

She didn't answer me right away. She looked thoughtful. I waited for her answer and thought how much I liked and trusted this woman. I had always felt a rapport with her, and many times she had proved her ability to treat the parent along with the child.

I remembered a long ago winter morning when Jonathan had just started walking. We were visiting a neighbor, and while she and I had coffee, our two toddlers played on the floor near us. Olene brought me a steaming cup and set it on the table. She returned to the kitchen to get one for herself. Furiously engrossed in gossip, I didn't see Jonathan heading for the table. With a mischievous baby giggle, he slapped his tiny hands on the table edge. But his fingertips caught the edge of the saucer instead. The plate and cup flipped backward toward Jonathan. Some incredible reflex caused me to grab the straps of his overalls from behind and jerk backward. The action made his chin tilt back so the coffee hit his neck and shoulder, with only a little splashing on his face. Otherwise he would have taken the whole cup of near-boiling liquid square in the face. The baby began to shriek and scream. Crying right along with him, I pulled his saturated T-shirt off his body because I knew it was continuing to burn him. A layer of skin came off his chest with the shirt, and I thought I might faint. My neighbor brought a blanket and wrapped my son in it. I picked him up and went to my car. Over my shoulder I called to her to phone Dr. Parrish.

Instinctively, I headed for Josephine Parrish. The hospital might have been a better choice, but I wasn't choosing, I was reacting. The baby continued to cry quietly during the ten-minute ride. With one hand I caressed his dark curls. He was so muffled in the blanket, I couldn't see most of his face. My beautiful son . . . if he were permanently scarred, I

8

would never forgive myself. And David would never forgive me either.

His perfect son. I remembered the excitement when he was born. Boys were at a premium in our family, and this one was welcomed jubilantly. When the obstetrician came out and announced to David and my father, "It has a Handle," there was pandemonium in the waiting room. Jonathan had been a source of his father's pride ever since.

Dr. Parrish was expecting us. She took my little bundle from me at the door and rushed down the hall to an examining room. She talked soothingly to Jonathan every moment, reassuring him and his mother at the same time. I realized I was still crying, but the baby had stopped. He only whimpered occasionally as she treated him, her hands so gentle and sure.

As she worked, I told her how the accident had happened.

"And now I suppose you're blaming yourself," she sighed.

"It was my fault. I should have been watching. I shouldn't have . . ."

"You are too intelligent a person to be thinking that way. You're worried about your husband, aren't you?" As I said— Josephine Parrish is an incredible lady.

"A little," I admitted, embarrassed. "He'll blame me."

"There is no blame here. Children get into accidents all the time. It's impossible to watch them every second, and it wouldn't be healthy even if it were possible. I'll speak to your husband myself." Dr. Parrish might have been a feminist long before it was popular.

"Now Sharon, some of these burns are second and third degree. Jonathan should be in the hospital." She spoke gently. She knew how I felt about hospitals. Jobi had been hospitalized with croup, dysentery, and a tonsillectomy, and the days I spent there with her had been an ordeal for me. I became horribly depressed even visiting someone in the hospital. The smells, the sounds, the sights in a hospital made me feel panicky. I had spent a long time in the hospital when I had polio as a very young child. I barely remembered it, but I often wondered if that experience was responsible for my present aversion to medical surroundings.

Dr. Parrish studied my dismayed face, and I could see her reaching a decision.

"I will teach you to care for him at home, but you should know it won't be easy." I listened with gratitude to her detailed instructions in caring for a burn victim. Jonathan recovered with only a few barely discernible scars, and I never forgot the sensitivity and personal concern our doctor had shown.

As I stood listening to Dr. Parrish's diagnosis of Jobi's trouble five years and many similar incidents later, I had no reason to doubt her.

"Jobi is the middle child," observed the doctor. "She's an easy-going, sunny child who is very undemanding. Isn't that right?"

"Well, yes."

"And I'll bet she's never taken as much of your time as Heidi or Jon."

"Dr. Parrish, Jonathan's the baby, and you know Heidi has always been a mittful."

"That's my point. Jobi's never been any trouble, and she hasn't gotten as much attention as the others. I think Jobi's demanding her time."

I was incredulous. "You mean you think Jobi's just pretending to have a pain in her knee?"

"The pain is real—to Jobi. But it's stemming from a need for attention; not an injury," Dr. Parrish stated firmly.

"It's hard to believe. It's so out of character for her."

She put her arm around my shoulders, and we walked toward the door. "Believe me," she promised. "You just take our little Jobi home and give her lots of T.L.C., and the pain will disappear." T.L.C. was Dr. Parrish's free prescription; a major part of any treatment. Tender Loving Care.

10

Jobi and I went home, and I thought over what I had learned. A tiny prickle went through me. I trusted Dr. Parrish completely. And yet . . .

I gave all the T.L.C. I knew how to give. Two weeks later, despite enough attention to have spoiled a Buddha, Jobi not only still had a pain in her knee, but a bad cold as well. She limped noticeably and was very quiet. There'd been no sunshine for days.

Even David, who was not one to use doctors unless absolutely necessary, agreed I should take Jobi back to see Dr. Parrish. I said it was because of the cold, but deep inside, the little prickle had never left.

The doctor prescribed a decongestant for Jobi's cold and X rays for her knee. "I still see nothing at all, but Jobi might feel better if the X rays show she's fine."

So might the mother, I thought, and we went to the outpatient department of the hospital and had routine X rays taken.

It was nearly dinner time when we got home, so I hurriedly settled Jobi back in her bed and filled her with decongestion medicine and children's throat lozenges. I went to the kitchen and began throwing pots and pans around with my usual inefficiency.

David came home, and I filled him in on our visit to the doctor and the subsequent X rays. "They'll let us know tomorrow or the next day," I concluded. He shrugged and asked what was for dinner. The mother's aide who lived with us set the table and got the other children ready for dinner.

The phone rang. Usually everyone ran at once to answer a ringing phone. But this time no one did. I dropped the pans with a clatter and reached for the demanding phone.

"Hello. This is Josephine Parrish."

How shall I describe what it felt like when my heart stopped for an instant? When movement around me froze and life hung suspended.

"Yes, doctor. " I hadn't been expecting the call. Had I?

11

"The X rays were unclear. They'd like you to bring Jobi back to have them retaken."

"All right. When tomorrow?"

"Tonight."

"I see. Why?" My voice was flat. It had no tone or cadence.

"Just routine, really. The X ray showed some . . . bony destruction and they'd just like to retake it." Her voice shook slightly. I remember thinking we knew each other too well for her to be playing this little game with me.

"Oh," I said lightly, all cheer and peanut brittle now. "Shall I bring pajamas or can she come right home?" The answer would tell me what I wanted to know.

"Oh . . . why not just bring the pajamas."

"Right. It can't hurt to have them there." We were soothing each other and beginning the motions of comfort.

I hung up and slowly sat on a chair. David came into the kitchen, scanning the newspaper headlines.

"Who was that?" he asked casually.

"Dr. Parrish." Something in my voice made him look up sharply. "They want to retake Jobi's X rays tonight."

"Tonight!"

"Yes. Now. Something about bony destruction."

"My God. Is that what she said?"

"Oh, it's just routine. Probably nothing."

"Probably nothing."

We wouldn't, couldn't look at each other. Woodenly, I went up to get Jobi. Passing Mary, our mother's aide, I gave her instructions for Heidi and Jonathan, who were watching television.

I entered Jobi's room. It was a different world from the rest of the house. We had lived in the spacious two-story home for two years, and I loved it as much as the day we decided to buy it. Each bedroom was decorated to suit the person who slept there. Jonathan's room was gold and avo-

12

cado, cheerful and warm, with happy toy soldiers marching across the wallpaper.

Heidi's room reflected her nature. I often thought of her as my little volcano—big for her age, but rosy and pretty with a will of iron and intelligence sparking from her eyes in warning flashes. When she was a baby, she trembled from head to toe if she became excited. Questioned about this, the doctor had just chuckled. "Some people have plow horses. What we have here is a thoroughbred race horse."

So Heidi's room was decorated in spicy coral with bright splashes of sassy tulips. It made me think of cinnamon ice cream.

Jobi's room was delicate pink with a canopy bed. Entering her room was like walking into a ball of cotton candy.

But I wasn't thinking of candy just then. I was thinking of Sunshine. She smiled when she saw me, her dimple flickering. I gathered her in my arms, color crayons and all. Then I tried to collect myself.

"Gotta get dressed, Sunshine. They messed up your X rays and want to take them over."

"Okay, Mom."

No questions, no arguments. Even when I packed her pajamas and robe in a bag, she showed little curiosity. Perhaps the decongestant had made her groggy. Or perhaps, like me, she knew.

4

ST. ANTHONY HOSPITAL. Wonderful modern facility where horrible things take place. White-clad, hard-faced people insisted Jobi go with them alone to have blood drawn and X rays taken. Jobi cried and begged me to come with her, but the hardfaces sternly said no. Later I would learn to deal with hardfaces.

When their poking and prodding had been completed, Jobi was assigned a room in pediatrics. There were few children on the floor so short a time before Thanksgiving, and the second bed in her room was empty. I helped Jobi into her pajamas while David glanced through a magazine. Neither of us knew what would happen next, and we were afraid to wonder too much about it.

Dr. Parrish entered the room followed by a man in a business suit. He was medium height, about thirty-five, with sandy, close-cropped hair. I had never seen him before.

"This is Dr. Pelletier," Dr. Parrish introduced us with a nervous smile. "He is an orthopedic surgeon." I couldn't hold back a soft gasp. David, his face pale, shook hands with Dr. Pelletier. We had not been expecting any other doctors, certainly not this rather cold-looking man.

"The X rays show something is definitely there," he said without preface.

"What? What's there?" I almost shouted. David grabbed my arm and nodded toward Jobi, who was coloring in a book behind us. We moved to the hall outside the room, everyone trying to appear casual.

"I don't know what it is," continued Dr. Pelletier. "It could be an infection in the bone, it could be a benign tumor, it could be anything."

"What are you planning to do?" asked David icily. I could see he was struggling for composure.

The doctor spoke curtly. "A biopsy tomorrow morning. Then we'll know better."

"What exactly does that mean?" I had trouble speaking. My tongue felt thick.

"We're going to do surgery on your daughter and see what's in there. If it's an infection, we'll treat it; if it's a benign tumor, we'll remove it. Then we'll have to take some

14

bone from somewhere else—probably the hip—to replace anything I have to remove."

I swallowed down vomit and clutched David. "If it's . . . something else?"

Dr. Pelletier stared at me for a moment before answering. "We'll talk about that then."

He nodded again and strode down the hall. I looked at Dr. Parrish. She reached her hand out slowly and placed it on my arm. "Eugene Pelletier is the best pediatric orthopedist I know."

I smiled weakly. She started to leave and then turned back. With a near sob in her voice, she blurted, "I didn't see it. I'm sorry. I missed it."

What could we reply? No one said anything for a moment. We stood there in the semidarkened hospital corridor. Somewhere, a baby cried.

"If a hundred children came to me with a sore knee, ninety-nine of them would be nothing."

"I know," I replied softly. I didn't blame her. David's face tightened. He said nothing.

We left Jobi there. She was tiny in the big bed. Her little rag doll, Mrs. Beasly, was cuddled in her arms. The original Mrs. Beasly doll was large, like the one in a popular television show of the time. My sister, Bonnie, had given Jobi a tiny version of the doll, with the same blue and white polka-dot cloth body and yellow yarn hair. Little Mrs. Beasly wore square wire glasses just like Jobi's, and my daughter decided they looked alike.

I kissed Jobi and she insisted I kiss her little cloth twin. David kissed Jobi too, but when she held up Mrs. Beasly, he pretended to gag at the thought. His antics made her giggle. As we walked away, I turned back for a moment. Jobi and Mrs. Beasly looked back at me with their blue eyes behind the wire glasses. Jobi smiled. Mrs. Beasly did not.

David and I spoke little that night. You can't talk if you're afraid to hear your own words.

15

I called my mother before I went to bed. I don't know what I said. I probably lied. I'm not sure why, but I had always felt my mother was the type of woman who needed to be protected from the grimmer things in life. She is very pretty and very young-looking, with thick blond hair, smooth clear skin, and fine classic features. David used to say he married me because he hoped I'd look like my mother when I grew old. Poor David. The only resemblance between my mother and me is our height. We're both about five two. But I have reddish fine hair, freckles, and my father's wavy nose. I enjoy dressing well, but have nowhere near the extent of my mother's love of beautiful clothes and need for all things to be pretty and matching. David thought she was flighty, and sometimes I agreed with him. We would both be proved wrong in the nightmare to come.

When I awoke the next morning, my teeth were chattering. I lay for a moment trying to ease my taut nerves. I swung my legs over the side of the bed and sat up. I looked at my legs. My left thigh is smaller than my right—a souvenir of the polio I had as a child—and the muscles are very weak. Sickeningly, it occurred to me I might have passed some physical defect on to my daughter. After all, could it be coincidence that polio had attacked my left leg and some unknown horror was attacking Jobi's left leg? Don't be ridiculous, I told myself. And then I prayed.

"Please God—don't let it be anything bad. I'll do anything. If bad things are meant for her—let them happen to me instead. Please . . . please . . ."

"I want breakfast," Jobi greeted me cheerfully.

"You can have breakfast later," I promised. "Remember? The nurse explained to you that before the doctor puts you to sleep, it's best not to eat or drink."

"Oh yeah," she answered, resigned. "Mrs. Beasly is going to be put to sleep too."

16

"Oh?"

"Uh-huh. I asked the nurse and she said she'd make 'rangements."

Just then a nurse entered. This was the smiling kind of nurse with a big needle on a tray.

"I have to give you a shot, Jo Beth. It will help you rest."

Jobi looked a little tearful, but she didn't protest. I held her hands while the shot was administered. A short time later, Grandma and Grandpa arrived and everyone pretended.

"Will it hurt, Mommy?" Jobi suddenly asked.

"No, love. You'll be fast asleep and you won't feel anything."

"Will you be there?"

"They won't let me come into the operating room with you, but when you wake up, I'll be right there. I promise."

David sat on the edge of the bed and joked with her until she got drowsy. "Mrs. Beasly's getting sleepy," she murmured.

With Mrs. Beasly tucked under her arm and a paper cap askew on her head, Jobi was pushed down the hall on a gurney by an orderly. She waved limply and the elevator doors closed in front of her.

My stomach lurched and I felt my jaws tightening. A sense of panic threatened to overwhelm me. But as I looked at the pale faces of my husband and my parents, I knew that for their sake I couldn't fall apart. Each of us was probably thinking the same thoughts, because as we sat in the waiting room, we all promised wonderful things to each other. And we talked about many subjects. Everything. Nothing.

David began to pace restlessly. He was never still or relaxed at any time, but that morning I could see he was fairly jumping out of his skin.

"Look," he said once. "It's just an infection or something. She's fine."

Everyone eagerly agreed. By now David's parents and a

few of my relatives had joined the waiting-room vigil. My large, boisterous family—aunts, uncles, cousins—rallied for blessed events and moments of crisis with equal fervor.

As I sat and waited, I didn't allow clear thoughts into my head. Specters and shadows lurked, but I firmly shoved them behind doors and held the doors shut.

So well did I rationalize, I was almost relaxed as David and I followed a woman, who was wearing a saccharine smile and a pink smock, down a corridor to a small room where, she said, "the doctor will come and talk to you."

We sat on a little couch. It was brown. It felt rough when I rested my hand on it. I could smell David's after-shave lotion as he sat next to me. It was spicy and it made me think of the first time I met him.

Freshman week at the University of Minnesota. A dance —somewhere. A tall boy came toward me. Crew cut, gray blazer with an emblem on the pocket, buff-colored half boots. Everything right. He put his arms around me as he said, "Dance?"

"It's cancer." I blinked for a moment at Eugene Pelletier in his green scrub suit. "It's a very rare cancer called osteogenic sarcoma." His lips were moving, but what was he saying? What was the matter with him? David's mouth opened, but nothing came out.

"We'll have to amputate her leg."

Then I saw that David's mouth was open because he was screaming, and I was screaming too.

Dr. Pelletier waited impassively, his face expressionless. A muscle in the doctor's check jumped slightly—the only sign he heard his own excruciating words.

"No!" cried David.

"You don't understand," I implored this green-clad stranger who spoke unspeakable evil. "It can't be Jobi. Everyone calls her Sunshine."

18

I don't think I fainted, but the memories are smudged. I didn't think I moved, but suddenly David and I were ushered into a chapel in the hospital. I saw someone run to the front of the small room where there was the image of a cross. Then a *Mogen Dovid,* the six-pointed Jewish star, was pulled down like a window shade over the cross. For a second I laughed at the nonsense.

A priest . . . minister . . . someone kindly but alien appeared.

"Go away!" I shouted. "Leave us alone!" Somehow the sight of the clerical-looking man infuriated me, made tragedy seem far too real. David just kept crying and crying. We put our arms around each other and cried like children.

My mother and my grandmother entered and came hurrying down the aisle of the chapel. I screamed, "Mom . . . Mom . . ."

"What is it? What's the matter?" Her voice was filled with terror.

"They're going to cut off her leg!" Now everyone was screaming and crying. Chaotic noise spread from the chapel to the corridor as hysterical aunts, uncles, and friends heard the ghastly news.

5

HOW DO YOU EXPLAIN to an eight-year-old girl that she is going to lose her leg the next morning? Neither David nor I was equal to that ordeal. Dr. Parrish, possibly in the grips of self-castigation, volunteered. The scene is seared in my memory.

I stood to the right of Jobi's bed, looking down at her

solemn, little-girl profile. It was dusk, and only one light was on behind me. David leaned against the door. Dr. Parrish sat on the edge of the bed. Jobi's leg was bandaged and propped on a pillow, so Dr. Parrish sat herself gingerly lest she disturb the wound. The woman took the child's hand in hers and looked into her eyes.

"Jobi, dear, I have something very important to talk to you about." I had to swallow repeatedly as Dr. Parrish spoke. "The doctor who operated on your leg found a bad thing growing there."

"How did it get there?" Jobi asked. "Is it because Ricky Kreiger kicked me?"

"We don't know for sure how it got there, dear, but if it stays, it could get bigger and hurt more than just your leg. So in order to stop it, the doctor has to take it away and everything around it."

"You mean I have to have another operation?" Tears blurred round blue eyes.

"Yes, sweety. You have to lose your leg. It's sort of like a barrel of shiny red apples and somewhere in the middle is a rotten one. If you don't remove the rotten one, pretty soon all the apples will be spoiled." Now Dr. Parrish was unable to stop the flow of tears from her own eyes. David turned and staggered into the hallway.

"Is it going to hurt me?" Jobi was crying.

"You'll be asleep, Sunshine. And you'll get a new leg almost as good as this one." This from me. Jobi considered the information.

"Will my new leg be on me when I wake up?"

Now I was crying and couldn't answer. Dr. Parrish responded gently, "The new leg won't be real, Jobi. But it will be almost like real and it will be made especially for you when you're home from the hospital."

Two women, each holding one hand of a small girl child. She looked at each of them and placed her trust and her life in those hands holding hers.

20

"Can Mrs. Beasly come with me?"

And Mrs. Beasly began her journey. The doll started the journey in a sterile plastic bag lying next to a sleeping child whose leg was amputated. The operation would later be described as L-AK: Left leg-Above Knee.

"I wish I could have left more," said Dr. Pelletier in his usual expressionless voice. We were in the same tiny room near surgery as the day before. My mind rejected what it could not accept. I hung suspended in a vacuum of unreality. My mother and David were shadows, the doctor a blotch. I didn't believe any of it was really happening. Certainly they hadn't removed my child's leg.

Dr. Pelletier continued, "I removed the leg four inches above the knee; as long as I dared leave it. I feel reasonably sure I got all of the tumor. But of course, the chances are still slim."

"Chances! Chances of what?" I stood up, his words snapping the world back into focus. David also stood. My mother, who had accompanied us today, didn't move. She just stared at the doctor.

"The chances that she'll live," he stated simply.

I wanted to kill him. Kill myself. And God died—at least for me.

"My whole family prayed for your daughter last night," he offered.

"I think you'd better explain what you said." David spoke calmly, but I saw the white around his mouth and the sweat beginning to trickle down his neck.

"Osteogenic sarcoma travels and reappears in the lung in ninety-seven to ninety-nine percent of the patients who have it." Dr. Pelletier said this without blinking.

I sank back onto the couch, and my mother and I began to cry quietly, leaning against each other. David covered his face with his hands.

Numb with shock and disbelief, a small dark thought flickered fleetingly through my mind. If we had known Jobi was likely to die in any case, would we have allowed the amputation to be done? Probably we would have made the same decision. The previous night we had called David's uncle, a prominent doctor from Hibbing, Minnesota, along with several other doctors we knew in Minneapolis. The answer was unanimous and definite—radical amputation was the only course of action for the rare tumor Jobi had contracted. But I couldn't help feeling bitter that we were not told it was almost hopeless from the beginning.

"You're telling us our child has only a one to three percent chance of living?" David gasped these words out.

"That's right. There is no treatment that has proven successful." The doctor seemed determined to hammer home the verdict. When I murmured inanely, "We were going to take the kids to Disneyland," Dr. Pelletier's rifle-shot reply was, "Do it. It's probably the last chance she'll get to see it."

How I hated him. The angry side of my sorrow turned full force against this blunt man. We later learned he was indeed an incredibly good surgeon. But his bedside manner was abominable. I had never before met such a negative, verbally brutal person. I was to meet many in the coming months.

"How long?" asked David.

"Six months to a year until the tumor metastasizes in a lung. After that . . ."

I stood for a moment in the doorway of the family waiting room. The faces I had known all my life looked up at me. No one moved or spoke. A frozen tableau.

There was my grandmother—my *bauby*—with thick silver hair and broad handsome face. Her heavy body was uncomfortable in the too-low couch. Her knotted hand clutched Marcia, her youngest daughter, who was perched on the arm of the couch next to her mother. My Aunt Marcia wore her counterfeit smile, and her arm was mottled where Bauby's fingers dug in. My other aunt, Charlene—not the oldest of

Bauby's five children, but the one with the power—stood with dignity next to her husband. Her face was without expression, but I sensed her fear. My mother and father had entered the room before me and stood to the side, his arm around her waist. Their grief-ravaged faces were composed now. In back of the others stood Edythe, David's mother. Her uncombed hair and smeared makeup bore witness to her stormy wait. Her piercing eyes bored into mine almost challengingly. Leonard, David's father, a short puffy man, remained seated, his face passive. I felt David's presence behind me, but he didn't touch me or speak. They were all waiting for me. I felt angry with them for making me talk. So I spoke angrily.

"Now look, I'm only going to say this once. I'll tell you what's happened so you understand. They did an above-knee . . . amputation." I gagged on the word, but went on. "They think they got it all, but the kind of tumor she has travels to the lung in ninety-seven percent of cases or more. They say she'll probably die, but we've made up our minds not to give up." I lowered my voice and leaned heavily on the words. "No one is going to quit. We will have hope. . . . We will remain in control. Jobi's going to live." I stopped for a moment, then challenged them, "Any one of you could get killed by a car tomorrow. Her chances aren't any worse than yours."

No one moved or spoke. I implored them. "Jobi is never going to know. You have to talk to your families. Make them understand that I need everyone's help so she won't know."

Those were all the words I had to give them. I started to sag. My father came up and put his arm around me, and Marcia ran up to me on my other side.

"I think she should have some coffee," Marcia said pointedly to my father.

"We'll take her," my mother spoke. I was numb and allowed myself to be led to the coffee shop. David was talking to his parents. It sounded like an argument,᾽ but at the moment I didn't care.

Marcia started to follow us down the hall, but Bauby called her back into the waiting room. I didn't see them again for a while. I later learned they had left the hospital. In the early winter snowstorm, Bauby and Marcia had gotten into Marcia's car and had driven through twenty miles of rush-hour, snow-laden traffic to the Jewish cemetery. They had ignored the wind and snow and walked to *Zady*'s grave. Zady, my incredible, almost biblical patriarch of a grandfather, had died the year before. Bauby needed to talk to him. They had been married for nearly fifty years. She had served and obeyed the dominating man most of her life. And now she had an order for him.

"Ike . . . Ike! Save her! You've got to help our Jobi."

It was a long time before Marcia could persuade the sobbing woman to leave her husband's snow-covered grave.

6

I DIDN'T LEAVE the hospital until the middle of the night. Jobi was in a pain-drug-induced stupor and I was a spaghetti person.

We entered our house. I crept into Heidi's room. I leaned down to kiss her forehead and saw she was sleeping with her glasses on. She must have tried to wait up for us. I removed the glasses carefully, and she stirred and muttered but didn't waken. I covered her. Little Jonathan slept the sleep of innocence. I leaned over his bed and sniffed the baby smell of his round cheek.

Silently David and I undressed and got into opposite sides

of our king-sized bed. We both lay staring into the night-filled room. Almost at the same moment, we both began to cry; the crying of two children who are frightened and lost. Then, with the primal instinct that is beyond all reason, we reached for each other's bodies. We could not kiss and feel and touch fast enough to satisfy the consuming passion that gripped us. Our need was greater that night than it had ever been, even when our love was new and beginning. And we made love nearly every night while Jobi was in the hospital. The cleansing, soothing, healing act of love was our only method of forgetting for a moment.

The first few days were a fog of pain for Jobi. She was drugged at all times, but it was never enough. She wouldn't let me out of her sight. Her tiny intensive care room became the center of my existence. I was so aware of her terrible need for my presence, I could hardly leave at night.

I awoke every morning with the same feelings. My stomach was hollow, my throat tight. I would sink into heavy gray and seek the night again.

And then I remembered Jobi and I thought I would die at the pain of it. My child of sunlight . . . reflection of my soul . . . and why, and why, and why?

Now get up. Wash. David has already left for work. Hurry. The other children need their mother too.

"Heidi dear, how about buying your lunch at school today and saving me some time? You don't like what they're having?" And inside I think, *But Heidi, I feel Jobi needing me. Please let me go.*

"Jonathan, did you brush your teeth?" *But if you get a cavity, Jon, I don't care because I have to go to Jobi now.*

They leave for school; I go upstairs to dress and make up carefully. Inside I feel a surging rush, but I control my hands and make myself pretty.

Since the first day of this nightmare, I had had a compulsion to look pretty. I didn't know why. In moments of the greatest inner agitation, I pulled out my makeup kit and applied lipstick or touched up my rouge. Visitors came to the hospital expecting to find a pale, tousled picture of an agonized mother. Instead they found a fashion plate. Did I think that if I looked good on the outside I would feel better within? I'm not sure.

The gifts began to arrive on the second day. From friends, relatives, neighbors, strangers. One hundred and forty-seven gifts, not counting pies, cakes, and even whole dinners left at our front door—often anonymously. People were determined to feed us and amuse Jobi . . . to sacrifice to the gods so such a calamity wouldn't happen to them.

Jobi's room was crammed with offerings. Stuffed animals, dolls, games, books. And flowers! Daisies and sweetheart roses in kitten-shaped vases, strawberry sodas that were really flower arrangements, and fluffy mounds of flowers that were really candy.

There arrived a ginger-colored stuffed dog named Henry who was taller than Jobi. Then came dolls who talked, walked, ate, wet, and even one who spit up. A little too realistic, the latter was removed from the collection. There was a complete set of Laura Ingalls Wilder's books, seven copies of *Charlotte's Web,* and four *Pippi Longstockings.* Jobi smiled and oohed and ahhed as the presents arrived, and Mrs. Beasly never left the crook of her arm.

Then a new world. A world without a leg. It meant buying pretty new pajamas for Jobi because she was in the hospital. Grandma brought them and everyone smiled. But we didn't know how to put them on. The stump was bandaged and sore, and no one wanted to tug pajama bottoms over it. I was dismayed, Auntie Marcia looked distraught, and Jobi was just plain disinterested. She didn't care about pajamas. She was worried someone would come in and do something to hurt her again.

Suddenly Grandma's eyes lit up. She left, carrying the pajamas, promising to return shortly.

A cheerful young man in a white shirt and pants arrived. He was pushing, of all things, a small pink wheelchair. Jobi eyed him with distrust.

"You must be Jo!" he bellowed, having a wonderful time. I winced. There was nothing that made Jobi angrier than to have people call her "Jo."

"My name is Jo Beth. Why are you here?" Jobi was never subtle; she always got straight to the point.

"Nothing to worry about, Mary Beth. You're just going for a little ride."

Jobi started to cry. "I don't want to go for a ride. It will hurt."

"Where are you taking her?" I asked timidly. Oh, what a long way I would come in the next few months.

"To P.T. They're going to teach Beth here how to walk on crutches." This information didn't sound too bad to me, but Jo—Mary Beth—Beth needed a little convincing. So I coaxed.

"Hey, Sunshine—you want to learn to walk around, don't you? You're going to feel really silly if I have to carry you down the aisle at your wedding." Little nasty thoughts crept into my head even as I said this. Little thoughts like "Who says she'll live to get married?" And, "Who's going to marry a girl without a leg?" But I mentally gave the thoughts a thwack and they disappeared.

With great care, the steadily chortling orderly lifted Jobi and placed her in the little wheelchair. She let out a yelp or two, but he had her seated and all tucked in under a blanket before she could protest further. I retrieved Mrs. Beasly from the floor, and our little group started down the hall.

Nurses and other parents smiled as we passed. I began to have visions of Jobi falling off crutches and breaking things; things like wrists, ribs . . . her other leg. So I didn't smile back.

Physical Therapy was very bright and sunny-looking. There were mirrors and bars and other shiny metal contraptions. There were tables with curtains around them and gym mats on the floor. A young woman with a chirpy voice greeted Jobi. She was the therapist who would be working with Jobi twice a day during her stay at the hospital. I was expected to attend since I had to learn how to wrap the stump in an Ace bandage and see that Jobi exercised it properly. I didn't even like the word *stump* and hadn't really looked at the stump yet. But I would manage. Of course.

A harness-type device was placed on Jobi, and two small crutches were brought. She was helped to stand by the young therapist. She felt a little dizzy and had to sit down again. But the second try was better. The crutches were adjusted, and Jobi was cautioned never to lean on them when they were under her armpits.

"Use your hands and arms, Jo Beth," said the chirpy therapist.

In an amazingly short time, Jobi was swinging along on the crutches. The therapist never let go of the harness and warned me to keep hold of it at all times until Jobi mastered walking on crutches. She allowed Jobi to take the crutches and harness back to her room so she could show them to her dad later. As one tired little girl was tucked back into her bed, Grandma returned, proudly displaying her invention. The crotch and inseam of one pajama leg had been opened and snaps sewn in. Now Jobi could snap and unsnap the pajama leg over her stump without hurting herself. Far-thinking Grandma had even given the same treatment to some little panties contributed by cousin Stacy.

7

THE THIRD MORNING after surgery, I was standing next to Jobi's bed holding a glass of Seven-Up. I knew she'd take only a sip or two, but even that small amount would help. She might have stopped eating and drinking altogether if I hadn't kept coaxing. And I knew the hideous intravenous unit couldn't be removed from her arm until she was drinking enough to prevent dehydration.

She allowed a small amount of the beverage to trickle into her mouth and listlessly pushed the glass away. Some of it spilled on her table and her gown, so I fetched some paper toweling from the bathroom and cleaned it up. It wasn't worth ringing for a nurse for something so minor, and I took care of as many of Jobi's needs myself as I could.

I threw the sodden mass of toweling into a wastepaper basket and picked up some other litter left in the room from the night before. A sudden feeling of weariness washed over me. I had the sensation that a plug had been pulled from my body and all my energy was draining like water from a bathtub.

I sank into one of the uncomfortable plastic chairs in Jobi's small room. It was like being buried in a sea of stuffed animals, dolls, and plants. I knew I was going to cry and wondered how I could leave the room so Jobi wouldn't see me.

An angel appeared—my mother. She burst cheerfully into the room, her blond hair beautifully coiffed, smooth skin glowing from the chill November air. The black mink coat she wore emitted a waft of flowery perfume.

I had a crazy urge to throw myself in her arms and say, "Mommy—help me—I can't do this." Even as the notion entered my mind, I thought how foolish it was. I was the strong one, not my mother. Ask anyone.

"Good morning, Sunshine," beamed the grandmother who looked more as though she should be the mother. "I brought you some new coloring books."

I looked at the stack of books my mother was displaying to an unresponsive Jobi. It didn't matter in the slightest to Helen Rosen that her granddaughter's room was already filled with coloring books, crossword puzzle books, and every other game book imaginable. She wouldn't dream of entering Jobi's room without bringing a gift, and she came on an average of twice a day.

My mother rose from kissing Jobi and scrutinized my face. "Sharon, why don't you go have some coffee?"

"No, I don't . . ."

"Rita is out there. I'm sure she'd like to visit with you before she comes in to see Jobi."

Only two people were allowed in the intensive care rooms at one time, and my good friend Rita Orensten would have to wait in the hall until either my mother or I left Jobi's room.

"Honey," my mother urged gently, "you look exhausted. You really need to leave this room for a little while."

"But, Mom, you know . . ." Wearily I indicated Jobi. My mother was aware how upset the child became when I left the room.

"I will stay with Jobi. We're going to have a nice game of ticktacktoe."

I was amazed at the firmness in her tone. She was such a gentle lady; assertiveness was alien to her nature. Also, I knew she was timid around illness and shrank from anything unpleasant.

"Go ahead," Mother insisted. Then with a bright smile at Jobi, "We'll be fine."

I knew my mother was right. I badly needed to leave the room for a while. I was numb with emotional fatigue, and my control was hanging by a fragile string. But I also knew she was not as confident about being alone with Jobi as she pretended. I was touched that she placed my need for a few moments respite above her natural fears.

I kissed my child and hurried out before she could protest. Rita greeted me warmly and squeezed my arm.

"How is she doing today?" she asked. I knew her concern was very real. My friendship with the tiny, doll-like woman had begun only a year before. She had appeared at the auditions of a new show I was directing for a community theater group. I took one look at her porcelain complexion and china blue eyes and cast her in the role of a child.

But while she looked as though she were about ten years old, Rita was anything but childlike. I discovered she possessed a keen mind, great sensitivity, and rare inner strength. We had been dear friends ever since.

Actually, we were another "Odd Couple." I was the typical haphazard housekeeper, so intent on the scene I was writing or the set I was designing that the house could have fallen down around me without my noticing. Rita, on the other hand, was a classic perfectionist. Her home was immaculate, her nails manicured, every strand of frosted blond hair in place. I once told her she should have been the one to marry David. They could have lived happily ever after in a sterile test tube. She laughed and agreed, except for one small problem—she and David couldn't stand one another.

Rita and I walked arm in arm to the elevator. "I dropped dinner off at your house on my way here," she mentioned. "I hope the kids like pot roast."

"You didn't have to do that," I protested.

"I don't have to do anything," she smiled. "I also threw in a load of clothes as long as I was there anyway."

I smiled at her affectionately. "You're really crazy, you know that." Only Rita would wash someone else's clothes—

31

not to mention the fact she did it despite the presence of the house girl whose job it was to do the wash. But I knew my friend's actions stemmed from an overwhelming need to help. While not everyone went to Rita's extreme, other friends and neighbors were reacting similarly. I rarely came home without finding a meal or cake someone had left.

We took the elevator to the main floor and sat at the counter in the coffee shop. Rita ordered a sweet roll and hot tea, but I opted for only black coffee. Food tasted like paste to me.

"Why aren't you eating something?" Rita scolded. "I'll bet you haven't had a bite to eat today." She called the waitress back. "Please bring my friend a toasted English muffin."

The waitress nodded and left. Rita turned back to me. "I know you like English muffins. You always ordered them at the deli after rehearsals."

"I'm afraid I don't like much of anything right now."

She was instantly sympathetic. "I know just how you feel; I remember how I felt when my mother was critically ill. Your stomach is in knots and your throat closes up when you try to swallow."

"You've got it," I agreed gloomily.

"But if you don't eat, you're going to get sick. Jobi needs you right now."

"I know that." I sighed and took a tentative bite of the muffin the waitress had just set down in front of me. It was lukewarm and soggy, but under Rita's sharp scrutiny, I managed to force down half.

"Sharon, my friend," continued Rita, delicately dabbing crumbs from her lips with the corner of her napkin, "no one ever said life was easy. This terrible thing has happened to your child, and you're angry. I don't blame you. But you have to consider the fact that Jobi is lucky. It might have already spread before they caught it."

"You know, Rita," I said bitterly. "Everyone keeps telling me how lucky she is. Well, can you tell me what in the hell is so lucky about getting cancer and having your leg taken off?" Now the flood of tears I had held back in Jobi's room could no longer be restrained. I sobbed from the depths of my soul, oblivious of the stares of other customers in the coffee shop.

Rita put her arms around me and let me cry as long as I needed to. When my sobs receded, she said, "I hear you, friend. I hear you. But my dear, she's alive. She is alive."

While this conversation took place, an even more dramatic scene was being played on the pediatric ward. I knew nothing of it until I returned less than forty-five minutes later.

After I left with Rita, my mother removed her coat and pulled a chair next to Jobi's bed. "Ready for ticktacktoe?" she asked.

Jobi smiled wanly and nodded. Within a short time, the child had won three games, and Grandma had finally coaxed a little laughter from her with desperate pleas for mercy in the next game.

"Jobi, I figured out that I've lost four hundred and thirty-seven dollars to you in the last two days. Grandpa's going to kill me."

Jobi giggled and, with mock cruelty, drew another ticktacktoe game. She made her X and tapped the paper impatiently, indicating her grandmother should hurry and take her turn. But Grandma was no longer looking at the game. Her eyes were on a figure in the doorway, and the smile slid from her face.

"Good morning, doctor," she said politely. Eugene Pelletier looked at her blankly. "I'm Jobi's grandmother, Helen Rosen." Her voice shook a little with nervousness. "We met the other day," she finished lamely.

"Oh yes. How are you? Jo Beth, how are you feeling?"

33

The child regarded him fearfully. His green surgical garb did nothing to reassure her. "I'm okay," she said in a barely audible tone.

"We're going to remove a few of those stitches," said the doctor, moving toward the bed.

"I want my mom," Jobi said, on the edge of tears. "Get my mom, Grandma."

"My daughter went to have coffee," said Helen tremulously. "I'll ask them to page her."

"That won't be necessary. I'm due back in surgery shortly, and this won't take long."

"But, doctor . . ."

"Nurse," Dr. Pelletier called. A nurse entered carrying a tray with the equipment he would need. He looked at my mother coolly. "Now, Mrs. Rosen, if you'll wait out in the hall, please. This will only take a few minutes."

Jobi began to cry. "At least let Grandma stay."

"Mrs. Rosen . . ." said the surgeon, indicating his impatience for her to leave.

My mother hesitated. She wasn't sure what to do. She had shared my dislike for Dr. Pelletier's manner, and the feeling was intensifying now into anger. She couldn't understand why it was necessary to cause the young child unnecessary anguish by forcing her to face this ordeal alone. But the doctor intimidated her greatly, and it took much courage to say, "Doctor, . . . Jobi would like me to stay in the room. I really think . . ."

"I'm sorry," the doctor snapped. "You'll have to wait in the hall."

Trembling with indignation and sorrow for her granddaughter, my mother surrendered and started for the door.

"Grandma! Grandma . . . please!" Jobi sobbed in terror.

Helen Rosen, embodiment of pliancy and vapidity, stopped in her tracks. She turned slowly back to the room, drew herself to her full five feet two inches of height, lifted her chin, and said, "Doctor—I am not leaving this room."

34

Doctor Pelletier looked at her with amazement, which quickly turned to annoyance. With a sigh of exasperation, he sat next to Jobi and began to remove her bandages.

Ignoring both his look and his sigh, my mother marched herself to the other side of the bed and held Jobi's hand, glaring at the doctor defiantly. Jobi's tears subsided, but she clutched her grandmother's hand tightly.

My mother could not restrain a soft gasp as the bandages were removed and the wound revealed. If Dr. Pelletier noticed, he gave no indication, but continued to work swiftly. Though Jobi cried out a few times as the stitches were removed, it was obvious even to my mother's inexpert eyes that the doctor had tremendous skill.

Nearly finished, he looked up at my mother's pale face. Her lips trembled as she used all her strength to keep from sobbing at her first sight of the stump. With a slight smirk, the doctor asked her to hold one end of the bandage while he brought the other end under the stump and back around.

My mother returned his gaze steadily, took a deep breath, and did as he asked.

The nurse quickly gathered the doctor's equipment and left the room. Pelletier started for the door, then turned back to look at my mother with reluctant respect.

"Mrs. Rosen, it was a pleasure working with you," he said with a slight mock bow. And Eugene Pelletier left the room.

8

THE WEEKEND WAS NO DIFFERENT from what the week had been, except the hospital was quieter and David stayed longer.

During the first few days my mind was too full of pain to realize something had changed between David and me. The quarreling and tension of the months before Jobi's illness had disappeared. Whether the truce was temporary or marked the beginning of a new and better relationship for us, I didn't know. For now it was enough that we had been drawn together during this time of trouble, rather than torn apart, as might have happened.

But these things were not on my mind as we walked through the sickeningly familiar hospital entrance on Saturday morning. As the elevator rose to the fourth floor, it was hard to believe only four days had passed since the beginning of this nightmare. It seemed as though it were years later, and I felt like an old woman.

David and I walked down the long corridor, heels clicking and making echoes. I suddenly became aware that David had taken my hand and held it firmly in his. It was almost a shock, albeit a welcome one.

David was not a handholder. Somewhere in his stormy childhood, an overbearing mother and temper-prone father had convinced him displays of emotion and affection were akin to weakness. One of the basic defects in our marriage occurred when my need for demonstrations of love met head-on with David's fear of giving it.

I looked up at my husband's face questioningly. He didn't

turn to look at me, but he gave my hand a little squeeze. I understood. Our almost frantic lovemaking of the last few days was instinctive and gave physical release and comfort. David's hand firmly enclosing mine was an emotional stroke; a promise to give whatever support I needed. I squeezed back.

David dropped my hand as we entered the pediatric intensive care unit. The nurse smiled and told us Jobi was asleep.

"I'm afraid she was pretty uncomfortable last night. She didn't get much sleep."

I knew "uncomfortable" was hospital talk for pain. But I pushed the rising heaviness in my chest aside so I wouldn't start crying for the hundredth time.

David and I walked quietly into our daughter's room. Her eyes were closed, dark lashes fanning pale cheeks. Her hair streamed wildly all over the pillow. I'd have to figure out a way to comb it soon, or the tangles would have to be cut out. Leaning down, I brushed her forehead gently with my lips so as not to waken her. David rarely kissed her or the other children, and he did not do so now. Instead he examined the intravenous bottle, its contents dripping steadily into the plastic tube leading to Jobi's tiny wrist.

His brief stint in premedical study as a youth had given him enough knowledge to have caused him alarm the day before. He had glanced at the intravenous unit and found it had stopped dripping. Something was clogging the line or the needle had slipped out of the vein. Either reason meant discomfort and possible danger to Jobi, whose skin was already becoming mottled and swollen at the needle site. David summoned a nurse, and the problem was easily dispatched. The nurse had explained she was scheduled to check Jobi in another moment or two anyway, so the child was never in danger. But David always scrutinized the intravenous unit when he entered the room after that.

Evidently he was satisfied that it was functioning properly, because he gave it a cursory check and came to stand behind me, his hand on my shoulder. We watched her for a few minutes, then David motioned for me to follow him back into the corridor.

"As long as she's sleeping, I'm going to run to the office for an hour or two," he said.

"Okay," I agreed. It was so difficult for David to remain confined in a room or to be forced to sit idly for any length of time.

"I'll be back later. I'll call you before I come in case you want anything." He kissed me briefly and strode back down the hall to the elevators.

I took off my coat and put it in a corner over a chair. Jobi stirred and opened her eyes. She moaned a little, but when she saw me, she produced a spindly smile.

"Hi, Sunshine."

"Hi."

I bent to kiss her, and she stroked my cheek with her free hand. "Hey, can I interest you in some fresh ice chips?"

"Uh-huh," she agreed. "I'm thirsty."

I was pleased with her response. She was reluctant to swallow anything, she had been feeling so ill since the surgery.

"Back in a jiffy," I promised. I had been given free access to the kitchenette where beverages, ice cream, and other refreshments were kept for the young patients. After the first day or two of apologizing to the busy nurses every time I requested something for Jobi, then waiting interminably until they had time to bring it, I finally asked permission to get things myself. The station nurse hesitated, then said, "Sure. Why not."

I scooped ice chips from a bin in the freezer and put them into a paper cup. Grabbing a plastic spoon, I hurried out the door, colliding with Dr. Parrish, who was passing the tiny kitchen at the same moment.

She laughed as she brushed ice chips off her dress, and I apologized.

Still smiling, she waved away my apology. "You're just the person I wanted to see." Josephine Parrish had been at the hospital two and even three times a day since Jobi's surgery. I knew one visit was her normal call on hospital patients. The other calls reflected her special involvement in the case and warm concern for all of us.

"There's someone I want you to meet," she continued, putting her arm around my waist and guiding me toward the nurses' station.

Seated behind the desk with his back to us, reading through a thick patient chart, was a gray-haired man in slacks and a sport jacket.

"Chuck?" Dr. Parrish announced our presence. "Sharon, meet Dr. Charles McMillan."

Dr. McMillan turned and, rising quickly, came from behind the desk to offer me a warm handshake. I couldn't help smiling back at the boyishly handsome face with flashing blue eyes under a shock of prematurely gray hair. He was a small man, about five feet eight inches, well dressed, if a bit unconservatively. I liked him immediately.

"Happy to meet you, Dr. McMillan," I said. I wasn't sure why Dr. Parrish was introducing us. My puzzlement must have shown, because she responded immediately.

"I wanted you to meet Dr. McMillan because he's a pediatric oncologist."

"Oncologist?" I had never heard the term.

"I'm a doctor for kids and I specialize in taking care of those with cancer," he said gently but firmly. "And that's the last time we'll use the word cancer because no one likes it very much."

I felt the lump rising in my throat and chest at his words. He could sure say that again.

"Sharon, I asked Dr. McMillan to discuss possible further treatment with you," said Dr. Parrish.

"Further treatment?" I said falteringly. Instant visions of giant machines shooting deadly rays into my small daughter . . . pictures of vile drugs being injected into her body. My teeth began to chatter as my jaw tensed.

"Let's go in the conference room," Dr. McMillan suggested.

"I . . . I have to bring this ice to Jobi," I protested weakly.

"I'll bring the ice to her," soothed Dr. Parrish. "I was on my way to see her anyway."

"But she . . ." I began to object.

"I'll stay with her until you're finished talking with Dr. McMillan," she added understandingly. I had to relent. I knew Jobi liked Dr. Parrish and would be happy enough in her company.

I smiled my thanks and allowed Dr. McMillan to propel me firmly down the hall to the conference room. I think he was afraid I'd change my mind about coming. He pulled out a bright-colored plastic chair, and I sat down tensely.

There was a coffee pot on a small table in the corner. Dr. McMillan poured two paper cups full and set one down in front of me. Sitting across the conference table from me, he sipped his coffee and made a face.

"I think they flavor it with Phisohex soap," he grimaced.

I tried to smile politely, but I was too nervous. I wished he'd get to the point.

He did. "I've studied Jobi's case, and I don't feel chemotherapy or radiation are called for at this time."

I looked at him with relief. "You mean you don't think she needs any more treatment?"

He chose his words carefully. "She should be watched very closely, of course. But I can find no evidence to support the use of chemotherapy, which means chemical treatment, or radiation therapy the way things stand. They just aren't effective in cases like this, so why put her through it?"

"I'm so glad to hear you say that, Dr. McMillan," I babbled, tears overflowing my eyes. "I was so afraid we'd have to subject her to more treatment, and she's been through so much already." Now my nose began to stream with my

40

eyes, and I realized I had left my purse—with Kleenex in it —back in Jobi's room.

Dr. McMillan gallantly produced a handkerchief and handed it to me. "Listen, you're welcome to get another opinion, or use another oncologist, for that matter."

"No," I blubbered, blowing and sniffling. "I want you."

"Okay," he grinned. "Let's go see that little gal of yours."

9

IT WAS SEVERAL WEEKS before David told me about his actions while I spoke with Dr. McMillan.

After leaving me at the hospital, David drove halfway to the office before he realized he had been driving by rote. Lost in thought, he scarcely remembered maneuvering through Highway 100's sluggish traffic in the light snowfall.

Wearily, he pushed his glasses up higher on the bridge of his nose and put on his signal light as he approached his exit ramp. There was a pile of neglected paperwork waiting on his desk. He had made only scattered calls on his clients in the last week, but fortunately, they were mostly old established customers of his family's packaging company. None of their accounts would be jeopardized by short-term neglect. Short term could grow to a long wait, however, if he effected the plan he had in mind.

After the first numbing moments when Dr. Pelletier had pronounced a death sentence on his daughter, David's mind began to rebel. He knew I was in no condition to plan beyond each day of torment, but he must think for both of us.

That thought process had begun shortly after I had taken Jobi to see Dr. Parrish the first time. Like me, David had

41

had trouble accepting the "middle child" theory as a diagnosis of Jobi's leg pain. But David's resistance to the idea stemmed from a different source than mine. While my introspective mind delved into the nature of our child, David's deductive nature explored a nagging, but elusive memory.

While a student at the University of Minnesota, David had maintained a part-time job as an orderly at Shriners Hospital for Crippled Children. For some reason, looking at Jobi's sore leg evoked a memory of that hospital where he had worked so long ago. There was no discernible mark on the leg, but a chill went through him. At first there was no connection. Then a scene emerged, and he remembered.

A young child was brought to the hospital one day—a six-year-old boy. He was crying, as many of them did at first. David overheard two doctors talking before he actually saw the child. They spoke in low tones, but he caught the words "cancer . . . surgery . . . little hope. . . ." He was asked to put the boy in a wheelchair and take him to a ward.

The young orderly pushed a small wheelchair into Admitting and scarcely flinched when he saw the child was an obviously recent amputee. One witnessed many sad, even bizarre sights working at Shriners Hospital, and David was no novice to assisting with these unfortunate children. He didn't see much of the little boy for the next few weeks. Then one day he learned the child had died. For some reason the news had great impact on him, though he had scarcely known the boy, and there had been other deaths while he worked at the hospital.

Looking at his daughter's leg, he had spoken in a cool voice to belie the horror he felt at the sudden memory of that little boy. He had said to me, "I think you'd better take her back to the doctor for another look." He had felt sure at that moment that Dr. Parrish was wrong.

Now, just a few days, but a seeming eon later, David was just as sure Dr. Pelletier was wrong. A man didn't just sit back and let himself be dumped on. He fought back.

Not that David had ever been much of a fighter. Over six feet tall in adulthood, he had told me often about the scrawny, undersized child he once had been. He was a favorite target of the Catholic boys who attended the parochial school near his home in St. Paul. They would wait for him to get off his school bus, then follow him, taunting and jeering.

"Sheeny!"

"Jew-boy!"

"We should pull down his pants and see if what they say is true."

"Ha—look at that scaredy-cat."

David would run as fast as he could to his house. The Catholic boys were much bigger than he, and they were right about one thing—he was afraid of them.

His father viewed the recurring incidents with disgust. "How can you let them pick on you like that? Stand up and fight like a man or you'll be running away all your life."

Finally his father's taunts made him angrier than the Catholic boys' taunts made him afraid. One day when the boys appeared at his bus stop in their matching uniforms, he took a deep breath and jumped on the boy nearest him. The small body knocked the bigger boy off balance, and they both fell to the ground. They rolled over and over, David pummeling his foe, tears streaming down his face. He got in a couple of good punches, and the other boy stopped struggling. In amazement, David looked down and realized he was sitting on his opponent's chest and had him pinned down.

"Do you give?" David asked as threateningly as possible.

The boy nodded. The rest of the gang hadn't moved or spoken, so astonished were they at the small boy's unexpected attack.

David climbed off the bigger boy, stood, and brushed off his hands triumphantly. His victim got up and looked at David warily for a moment.

43

"So there!" David couldn't help adding. And suddenly a fist smashed into his face, knocking him to the ground.

"So there yourself," said the older boy calmly, and he and his buddies walked away.

David got up and brushed the tears from his eyes. Dragging his feet, he started for home. But as he walked, he began to straighten his shoulders and walk more briskly. Then a grin began to spread across his grimy, tear stained face.

"I fought him," he thought. "At least I fought him." And the Catholic boys never bothered him again.

David's thoughts were on a fight of a different nature as he parked his car in the spot reserved for him as sales manager and entered the new building that housed the packaging plant. The office section was at the front of the long low structure, and the receptionist said there was a call for him as he passed her desk.

He went to his cubbyhole office and picked up the receiver. "Oh—hi," he said. It was his mother calling to check on Jobi's condition. Edythe and I did not get along well, and his mother generally called him rather than me.

They discussed Jobi and the other two children for a few minutes. Edythe expressed her fears that Heidi was feeling neglected during the last few days. Of the three grandchildren, it was Heidi she had always been closest to, possibly because Heidi had been the first. David agreed that indeed both Heidi and Jon were feeling a little neglected, but he didn't see what could be done about it at the moment.

Abruptly, David changed the subject. "Isn't there a cancer research center somewhere near where Diane lives?" he asked. Diane was his married sister who lived in Maryland.

"Yes, but I can't think of the name of it. Why don't you call Diane?"

"I think I will."

"What do you have in mind, son?"

"I can't just sit and wait, Mom. I've got to do something."

"I know. Go ahead—call Diane."

44

David hesitated for a moment after putting down the receiver. He wasn't sure what path he was taking or what he expected to do with the name of a cancer research center in Maryland. But placed the call.

Diane supplied him with a name—Bethesda—and the telephone number listed in her directory.

He heard the phone ringing . . . three, then four times. A crisp female voice answered.

"Bethesda Medical Center."

"Hello. I'd like to speak to one of your doctors involved in cancer research," David blurted uncertainly.

The switchboard operator hesitated, then snapped, "And who may I say is calling?"

David could tell by the haughty tone of her voice that he didn't stand a chance of reaching one of the great medical deities if he were plain old David Nobody of Minneapolis. He chose a mild subterfuge and silently prayed it would work.

Dropping his voice to what seemed like an official, commanding tone, he said, "This is David Halper calling from Minnesota." He hoped Minnesota would summon connection in the receptionist's mind with the Mayo Clinic in Rochester, Minnesota. "I have a patient here with a rare case of osteogenic sarcoma. Now young woman, are you going to connect me with the proper person or not?"

The cool voice changed and became ingratiating. "Oh, of course, Dr. Halper. I'll put you through to Dr. Bearing at once."

She clicked off. David felt in his pocket for a handkerchief. He always perspired freely, and now sweat was pouring down his neck.

Dr. Bearing came to the phone. With little preamble, he told "Dr." Halper that while little was being done at Bethesda on osteo, his best best was to get the patient into a protocol study.

David didn't want Dr. Bearing to know he hadn't the foggiest notion what "protocol study" meant, so he quickly asked, "Do you know where there's a protocol study at present?" He hoped he had used the phrase correctly and not given himself away.

If there was anything amiss, Dr. Bearing appeared not to notice. He answered, "Well, I'll tell you, no one has very many osteo cases. But Roswell Park in New York is dealing in something similar, and you could try St. Judes . . . no, I think they're strictly leukemia. Stanford comes to my mind, and of course, M. D. Anderson at Houston is always into something."

David decided to push his luck all the way and ask Dr. Bearing for specific names to contact in the various medical centers. Bearing supplied the information readily, and David decided to quit while he was ahead. He was half afraid the doctor would ask him a question, and he knew he could never bluff through a medically oriented answer.

His fear was realized. Before he could end the call, Dr. Bearing said, "I take it you fellows at Mayo are still using mainly cobalt."

"Uh—yes. Cobalt."

"Well, I'll be honest. I don't think it's worth much. But then, no one has an answer for sure, do they?"

"No, I guess not. Thank you for your help, Dr. Bearing."

"That's all right. And good luck."

David put the receiver down in relief and leaned back in his chair. He had done it. He had bluffed his way through the call. And he knew he would do it again. He would call every name on the list Bearing had given him, and he hoped to be able to add others as he went along.

He looked at his watch. It was too late to make any more calls today. It was sheer luck he had found someone in at Bethesda on a Saturday morning. But Monday, he decided, "Dr. Halper" would be on the line again.

10

I LEARNED LATER that David decided to wait before saying anything to me or anyone else about his calls. He felt it was pointless to discuss or argue about it until he had all the information he required.

In his typically methodical manner, David had stopped on his way back to the hospital to purchase some file cards. On these would go names, places, and protocol studies for later perusal. He reminded himself to find out exactly what "protocol study" meant before he made any further calls.

Returning to Jobi's room, David passed Dr. Parrish, who was leaving. She smiled at him tentatively, and he responded with a curt nod. Their relationship had become strained to its limits since the day she had admitted to missing a diagnosis. It wasn't that he held her responsible, but being a perfectionist himself, he expected no less from those around him. While he liked Josephine Parrish personally, I knew he could not forgive what he considered to be a professional weakness.

Jobi was awake and smiled happily when she saw him. After my talk with Rita, even I felt more relaxed than when he had left a few hours earlier.

A nurse entered to take Jobi's blood pressure, pulse, and temperature. This activity never disturbed her, so I took advantage of the distraction to lead David out into the hall. I related my meeting with Dr. McMillan.

Weeks later David told me that he had felt his heart sink as he listened to my recital of the new doctor's opinion. I was obviously very impressed with Dr. McMillan. He had wondered how he was going to fight my reluctance to subject

Jobi to further treatment if I was fortified by a professional.

"I can't wait for you to meet Dr. McMillan, David," I said enthusiastically. "He's so nice and understanding. And you should have seen him with Jobi. He had her laughing and playing two minutes after he walked in her room. It was the first time she wasn't afraid of a doctor. Come to think of it, it was the first time she's laughed."

Then David realized the situation would be even more difficult than he had anticipated. If what I said was true, this Dr. McMillan had both his wife and daughter mesmerized. He steeled himself to keep from showing his annoyance at the doctor's interference.

"Well, I can't wait to meet this paragon." He tried to smile, realizing his tone had been more sarcastic than he intended. I looked at him in surprise, then decided to ignore the barb.

We returned to Jobi's room and neither of us mentioned Dr. McMillan for the rest of the afternoon.

11

DR. PARRISH THOUGHT it would be a good idea if Jonathan and Heidi came to the hospital to visit their sister.

They had eagerly clamored for news of her each day. They drew pictures and made little gifts. I thought they'd be very excited when they learned they could actually see Jobi.

But they weren't. I told them Dr. Parrish was making special arrangements so they could be admitted to the fourth floor. I explained that normally a little boy of five and a girl of ten weren't allowed to visit patients. But a special exception was being made in their case.

The two children grew very quiet. The flurry of questions and exclamations I had expected didn't occur. They wouldn't meet my eyes.

"Heidi . . . Jon . . . you want to go, don't you?"

Jonathan finally looked up at me, his dark eyes troubled. He saw that he was disappointing me by his lack of reaction and tried to make up for it.

In an artificially cheerful tone I wouldn't have thought a five-year-old capable of, he said, "Oh boy—yeah—we get to see Jobi!" Then his face darkened, and in a fearful voice, he asked, "What does she look like now?"

"She looks just like she's always looked, Jon," I reassured him.

"She does?" he asked doubtfully.

"Of course." I turned to my daughter. "Heidi . . . ?"

Heidi still hadn't looked at me. Suddenly she whirled around and said defiantly, "I'll go see her . . . if I don't have to touch her."

Then I realized how terrified my children must have been all week. I thought they were too young to react the same as the rest of us. They had been given a watered-down explanation of what had befallen their sister in an attempt to protect them. All we had succeeded in doing by screening them from reality was to frighten them more. With little information at their disposal, their fear of the unknown had done more damage than the facts might have done.

And how could I blame these children for being reluctant to see Jobi? I could hardly look at her myself the first time. I struggled for the right words.

"Kids, listen . . . we all know it's a terrible thing that Jobi had to lose her leg. But it saved her life.

"Now she has only one leg, but in every other way she's the same sister you've always had. Of course, she'll need our help more than she used to, but we won't mind because we love her."

Jonathan was nodding gravely; Heidi's expression was

unreadable. I could tell they needed more, so I continued.

"You shouldn't be ashamed of being afraid to see Jobi. I was a little afraid myself the first time."

"Oh, sure," scoffed Heidi. She recognized a soothing speech when she heard one.

I ignored her comment. "But there really isn't anything to be afraid of. Within a few minutes, you'll see it's our same old Jobi."

"Where do they keep her in the hopsible?" asked little Jonathan, unaware he had mispronounced the word.

I smiled and drew him onto my lap. "Jobi has a nice big bed in her own little room, Jonny. But when you see her, she'll be in a wheelchair." I raised my head to include Heidi, who was looking out the bay window.

"Heidi, you and Jonathan will come up to the fourth floor lounge, and I'll bring Jobi out to see you. There's more room there, and we'll all be more comfortable."

Heidi was quiet for a minute or two, then she said, "Fine," and went up the stairs to her room.

I decided there was nothing more I could say for the moment. I felt sure they'd lose their apprehension once they saw Jobi.

12

WHEN YOU CAN'T DEAL with a giant problem, it becomes necessary to tackle one your own size. My mother and I decided to wash Jobi's hair in honor of her brother and sister's expected visit. It was a formidable decision.

Long, thick, silky hair that is lain upon for a week becomes a tangled bird's nest. For the untangling ceremonies, I produced two sturdy brushes; one for me and one for my mother. We approached the target hesitantly, brushes raised.

The owner of the bird's nest eyed us warily. "What are you going to do?" She used a warning tone. In her opinion, her hair was just fine.

"We're going to brush your hair out and wash it?" My sentence had started out firmly, but my voice rose in doubt as I saw a scowl mar the small brow.

"How come?" she demanded.

"Your hair looks as if it lost a fight with a Mixmaster," my mother offered hopefully. Jobi looked unconvinced.

"I think I saw a bug crawl out of it," I said evilly.

"Where?" Jobi asked, weakening. I closed in.

"If we can't brush it out, we'll have to cut it short."

"Brush." She surrendered.

Our backup unit, the intensive care nurse, rolled in a gurney and lifted Jobi onto it with ease.

"What's this?" Jobi asked, apprehensive again.

"Your beauty shop," I explained. I pulled all her hair backward so it hung down over the edge of the gurney. My mother and I sat in chairs behind her and each took a matted strand.

"Whoo!" I expressed my feelings toward the challenge facing us.

"You can say that again," agreed my mother.

"Don't hurt me," ordered Jobi.

"My dear," I philosophized. "It hurts to be beautiful."

It took the better part of an hour to brush the hair smooth enough to consider washing. Then we pushed the gurney into the corridor where there was a utility sink.

Armed with guaranteed tearless shampoo and a spray bottle that promised to "Untangle Snarls Effortlessly," we washed Jobi's flowing mop.

She was tearless. I was not. Suds and water splattered

everywhere. My pushed-up blouse sleeves kept falling down into the water. My mother had blobs of suds dotting her face. The floor was slippery and free from tangles.

Jobi, a pleasant smile on her face, lay unconcerned as we slaved over her hair. She enjoyed herself thoroughly.

Later, as she sat propped up on her pillows, her hair cascading gloriously around her shoulders, I looked over at my mother and started to laugh. She looked back at me indignantly, then began to laugh even harder. We both resembled victims of a rogue washing machine; sodden clothing, hair hanging limply, makeup smeared.

Jobi patted her clean, shining hair smugly. "Boy, you guys look terrible. You should comb your hair or something."

13

DAVID WAS DUE TO BRING Heidi and Jonathan to the hospital at six-thirty. At six, Jobi began to fret and complain her tummy hurt. Oh no, not now, I begged her silently. I wanted Heidi and Jon's first visit with their sister to go well.

"Let me brush your hair and get the little pink wheelchair," I suggested as cheerfully as possible. "Maybe by then you'll be feeling better."

"No, Mom. I feel icky."

"Sunshine, I know you aren't feeling terrific, but Heidi and Jonathan are on their way here. They're looking forward to seeing you."

"Okay," she said with a sigh.

I fetched the wheelchair, and as I returned to the room, Jobi was crying softly.

"Honey, what is it?" I gathered her in my arms.

"Mom, it's my foot. It feels like someone is taking my toes and bending them backward."

I leaned over and lifted the sheet off her slender foot. "It looks okay, Jobi, maybe . . ."

"Mom, not that foot."

I didn't know what to say. Was she delirious? She didn't have another foot. We just stared at one another. Tears rolled down both our faces.

Suddenly, Jobi wiped her eyes with a piece of tissue from the box on her nightstand. Then she took another piece and tried to wipe mine. "It's okay, Mom. Don't cry. It stopped hurting now."

I hugged her tightly. Love and anguish swelled inside my chest.

"Hey," she protested. "You're squishing me."

I managed a laugh. "That's because you're so squishable."

David appeared in the doorway. "We're here," he announced.

"We're almost ready," I said. "Why don't you wait with the kids, and I'll bring Jobi in a minute."

He looked from my face to Jobi's questioningly. I shook my head slightly to indicate he shouldn't say anything more.

"All right. Hurry it up, girls."

I put Jobi's bathrobe on her and lifted her into the wheelchair. It was easy, her body seemed weightless. I tucked a blanket around her lap, careful that the fact that her leg was missing was indiscernible. The visit would be hard enough on Heidi and Jonathan without any immediate shocking sights. There'd be time enough for that later.

I wheeled Jobi to the lounge. She slumped in the chair, her face very white. I knew she was feeling pain again, but real or imagined, I couldn't guess.

The children were full of constraint. It was obvious none of them knew what to say or do. Jonathan looked very frightened, and Heidi kept staring at Jobi's blanketed lap.

David and I made small talk, trying to put them at ease, but it was futile.

"Jonny, why don't you tell Jobi about what you found in the backyard?" I suggested brightly. When you have to tell your kids what to say to each other, you've had it.

Poor Jonathan looked at me blankly for a minute. Then, in a shy monotone, "Oh yeah—I found a baby mouse. But I couldn't keep it."

Jobi smiled wanly. Another silence ensued.

"When is she coming home?" asked Heidi, as though her sister weren't in the room. "For Thanksgiving?"

"We don't know yet, honey," I answered. I had the feeling she was hoping it would be more like next spring some time.

"Mom, can I go back to my room now? I don't feel good." Jobi drooped languidly.

"Of course, Sunshine. Heidi and Jonathan can come back another time." I was lying and everyone knew it. The visit had been a dismal failure, and no one was interested in a repeat. I only hoped the fear and tension would disappear when they were all home in familiar surroundings.

David told Heidi and Jonathan he would be right back, and accompanied me as I pushed Jobi back to her room. I looked at him sadly, and he put his arm around me.

As David lifted Jobi into bed, she gasped and started to cry.

"Did I bump your incision, Jobi? I'm sorry!"

"No—no, Daddy. . . . It's my foot. Oh, it hurts. It's like a car is running over it."

As I had done earlier, he reached for her foot to see why it hurt. I stopped him.

"She doesn't mean that foot, David."

"What?"

"This happened earlier."

Awareness dawned on his face. "I see."

54

"Should we call the doctor in?"

"We don't have to. Pelletier told me it could happen, but he was hoping it wouldn't because she's so young."

"What are you talking about?"

"Phantom pains. It happens to amputees. The brain doesn't accept the loss of the limb, and keeps sending signals."

"My God."

Jobi cried out, and I put my arms around her. New anguish filled me. How much more could we withstand, Jobi, David, and me? I found out later. More . . . much more.

14

JOBI HAD BEGGED to go home for Thanksgiving, but her doctors agreed it was too soon.

Reluctantly, we left her for an hour or two on Thanksgiving day. My family, thirty-two kinfolk strong, was having dinner together and had persuaded David and me to join them. We agreed because Heidi and Jonathan looked so forlorn when we said we might not go this year.

I scarcely ate, as opulent platters enticed everyone else into their usual eating orgy. I felt removed from the chatter of familiar voices and tinkle of silverware and china. I had no body, and my mind floated above the long row of end-to-end tables. The room seemed shadowy, but now and then a face was illuminated for an instant.

There was Aunt Charlene, busy directing the flow of tray traffic. Affectionately, I envisioned her in a police uniform. I almost heard her blow a whistle when someone lingered too long over a platter of steaming *varnishkes*—

buckwheat groats fried in chicken fat and mixed with pasta.

My two young sisters, Leenie and Bonnie, sat at one end of the table with the college-age cousins. Their nearly matching pretty faces glowed as they laughed and sipped Mogen David wine. Larry, my handsome bachelor brother, flirted with all the girl cousins. He liked to keep warmed up in case the real thing came along.

A fragmented piece of my mind overhead David and Aunt Marcia, who were deep in discussion. But I picked up phrases like . . . "friend of mine who had cancer . . ." ". . . they gave her up . . ." ". . . went to Houston . . ." I snatched my mind away from them.

My dear Bauby called to me. "Eat! You're getting too thin!" How I loved her. When I was nine months pregnant, she thought I was too thin.

My father's eyes met mine. The depth of his sadness clutched at my throat. His compassion reached out and enveloped me in a heavy blanket.

I had to leave. The presence of tragedy hung above the table where my mind floated. Everyone laughed and pretended nothing was wrong. For some of them, there was no pretense—the young don't dwell on sorrow.

"David," I whispered. "Please, let's go."

He nodded and pushed his chair away from the table. He, too, had had enough. Suddenly, the warm, cheerful atmosphere seemed almost obscene.

My aunts scurried about and produced a bulging package of food we were to bring to Jobi. She wouldn't eat it, but they needed to give of themselves, so I accepted their gift.

My parents would bring Jonathan and Heidi home, so David and I returned to the hospital. To Jobi. During the ten-minute car ride, Thanksgiving made me cry.

15

JOBI CAME HOME. It took four cars to get her there. One held Jobi, my mother, Mrs. Beasly, and me. David's station wagon overflowed with stuffed animals and toys. Also a wheelchair. My father was the traveling florist—plants threatened to engulf him as he followed David's car. Rita brought up the rear of the caravan, transporting miscellaneous items that didn't fit anywhere else.

"Welcome Home Jobi" signs festooned the entry to the house. Jobi giggled when she saw them. The small artists responsible for the display peered anxiously through the bay window.

David pulled in behind me in the driveway and began taking out the collapsible wheelchair we had rented. But Jobi had other plans.

"Give me my crutches. I can walk."

My mother started to protest, but I motioned her to silence. I pulled the crutches from the backseat and brought them to Jobi. They were painted a shocking pink and were decorated with brightly colored flowers and butterflies. A friend from one of my theater groups had brought paints and brushes to the hospital one day, and we helped Jobi create the incredible-looking crutches.

My heart clogged my throat as I followed the slight child toward the front door. There was a thin layer of snow on the sidewalk, and she left behind a trail of one bootmark with two crutch-tip indentations slightly ahead of it.

The short walk used up her small energy reserve, and she lay gratefully back on the couch in the family room. But there was a triumphant twinkle in her eye.

As David, my parents, and Rita unloaded the cars, I went into the kitchen to make coffee. I heard the three children chattering away as if nothing had ever happened.

Nothing had ever happened.

I came back into the family room in time to see Jobi displaying the stump of her leg to a fascinated Heidi and Jonathan. The ordeal I had most dreaded had been dispatched quickly and painlessly by my resilient children. They looked at the healing wound, expressed proper respect, and turned the television set on to a Walt Disney program.

A routine established itself in the week that followed. Each morning David carried Jobi down the stairs and deposited her on the family-room couch. She would soon be flying up and down those stairs on her pink crutches, but it would take a little more time for that kind of strength to build.

Heidi and Jonathan ate breakfast with their sister before they went to school. David never ate breakfast, and he left hurriedly each morning. He seemed preoccupied, but I hadn't the energy to worry about it. We were still being very soft with each other, and I was content.

People visited all day long. I began to appreciate the stacks of cakes, pies, and cookies that had accumulated in my freezer—donations from weeks past. Guests visiting the sick like to be fed.

One afternoon, three little girls came to the door. They each bore a little wrapped package, and they smiled shyly. I recognized them as friends of Jobi's who attended Olson School with her. They all lived nearby and played together often.

"Can we see Jobi?" piped up the bravest. It was Cheryl Friedman, brown eyes snapping.

"We have presents for her," added Judy Sher. Her rosy, freckled face dimpled. The third child, Julie Shwantes, had moved to the neighborhood recently. She was very shy and kept her eyes on the ground.

"Of course you can visit Jobi," I welcomed them. "She'll be so happy to see you."

And she was. She had been fretful with phantom pains most of the day, but they disappeared magically when she saw her friends. They chattered like magpies for the next few hours, devouring plates of Hydrox cookies and a half gallon of milk.

The first call from a polite mother requesting the return of her child broke up the party. They left regretfully, promising to return often. And they kept their promise. At least one of the little girls came over every day.

They didn't realize it, but the visits of these and other children would pull Jobi back from the abyss of chemical-induced horror. But that was later.

16

MEMORIES OF WEEKS that followed . . . a kaleidoscope of flashing scenes.

A few days after Jobi's homecoming. My neighbor, Jeanette Glimmerveen calls and tells me she and her family have formulated a plan. She explains what they want to do. I try to protest, but she is adamant. The next night we celebrate a real Thanksgiving . . . all of us together. The Glimmerveens, Jeanette, John, and their handsome sons, Mark and Doug, are providing Thanksgiving dinner for the Halper family. Jeanette, wielding a turkey baster, does the cooking. John, a towel over his arm, acts as waiter complete with many bows and a great deal of heel clicking. Mark and Doug are the busboys, grins plastered on their faces. We all laugh copiously and eat even more.

Jobi's teacher, Ann Cheleen. One of those rarities we call a fine human being. I throw her a curve, and instead of being confounded, she catches it and runs.

Jobi's stump has to be wrapped in an Ace bandage at all times. The bandage has to be rewrapped several times a day in a prescribed manner. In addition to this, there are certain exercises Jobi must do three times a day that require some assistance. One of the three times falls at midday during school hours. While none of this is difficult, it isn't the most pleasant of tasks for a novice. But someone has to do it, or Jobi can't go to school.

I discuss the situation with Ann Cheleen on the phone. I wonder aloud if it would be practical for me to try coming to the school several times a day; or could the health aide at Olson help?

"Don't worry, Mrs. Halper. I can do it," says the pleasant teacher.

"Oh no, we couldn't ask that of you. You have your hands full just dealing with thirty eight-year-olds."

"Please—I insist. I want to do it."

She finally persuades me to let her try it for a few days. If it doesn't work out . . . well, we'll wait and see.

We later learn Ann Cheleen was a volunteer at St. Anthony Hospital. While not wishing to intrude in our personal crisis, she had been a silent observer to those first hellish days.

"I was crying too," she tells me.

Jobi's first day back to school. I don't think she's ready,

but Jobi and her friend Dr. McMillan convince me I'm the one who isn't ready. Jobi will do just fine.

She wears a long red wool skirt . . . a gift from Grandma Helen. I think how lucky we are that long skirts and dresses are in style for daytime wear, even for children. I tie bright red ribbons in her hair, and she ties matching ribbons on her crutches.

Everyone knows she's coming, and when we pull up in front of the school, her teacher, the principal, and most of her classmates are outside to greet her. Eager hands help her from the car and set up the collapsible wheelchair. She still tires easily on the crutches, and though she dislikes the chair, it must accompany her.

The children clamor for the privilege of pushing the chair. But the lucky boy chosen pushes an empty one. As I could have predicted, Jobi chooses to walk into school with her crutches. She swings up the walk, heedless of the slush, surrounded by her excited friends. Jobi is a celebrity.

A Saturday morning. David has taken Jonathan with him to the office. I sit at the kitchen table making notes on a script. The kitchen opens onto the family room where Jobi and Heidi simultaneously play ticktacktoe and watch television. Both girls wear flannel pajamas and quilted bathrobes; both have their dark blond hair caught in pigtails. Their wire-frame glasses are similar, and so are the expressions of concentration on their faces. They probably wouldn't like to hear it, but they look very much like sisters.

"There—'X'—I beat you," says Jobi triumphantly.

"That's because everybody plays with you all the time, and you get a lot of practice," replies her disgruntled older sister.

"You can pick the next show we watch," Jobi offers contritely.

"No," says Heidi, standing up. "I'm gonna get dressed and go over to Lisa Plitman's house."

61

"But I thought you don't like Lisa," says Jobi in a disappointed tone to Heidi's retreating back.

Heidi turns and looks at her coldly. The unspoken message hangs in the air above them. "I don't like you very much either."

Our trip to Dr. Pelletier's office. The rest of Jobi's stitches need to be removed. David leaves work to accompany us.

The orthopedic surgeon greets us in his usual cool manner, doing nothing to put a frightened Jobi at ease. By this time, the very sight of the man makes my blood run cold.

He dispatches the remaining stitches deftly. No one could ever question his medical skill. David jokes with Jobi, trying to take her mind off the stinging sensation as threads are snipped.

While I'm helping Jobi up from the table she is lying on, Dr. Pelletier says offhandedly, "That stump is quite cone shaped. If the bone gets too long, the end of it will have to be taken off later."

I stand frozen with shock and horror at his words. How could he say such a thing in front of Jobi? It is monstrous.

Jobi begins to hiccup and give little gasping sobs. I put my arms around her; her small body is trembling. David stares at Pelletier. The veins stand out on his neck. I think he might hit the doctor. Instead, he picks Jobi up and strides out of the room. I grab her crutches and hurry after him. We never see the obtuse Dr. Pelletier again.

17

FOUR WEEKS AFTER Jobi's surgery, it was time for a checkup by Dr. McMillan and her first chest X ray. Since the lung is the usual target area of osteogenic sarcoma, monthly chest X rays are mandatory.

While Dr. Parrish was still officially Jobi's pediatrician, for the present, Dr. McMillan would take care of her. I took her to his office after school. We entered the bright waiting room, and several people turned to stare at Jobi's pinned up pant leg. I felt embarrassed, ashamed of my embarrassment, and angry at the people all at the same time. Jobi appeared not to notice. She swung cheerfully on her crutches into the waiting room and plopped on a chair. She wasn't afraid of this visit to the doctor. Charles McMillan was her friend.

"Well . . . it's the Halper girls," Dr. McMillan teased, entering the small examining room. Jobi giggled.

"Laughing, eh? I'll bet you think it's funny that I'm working and slaving while you lie there on that nice soft table."

Jobi giggled again. "This table isn't soft—it's hard as a rock."

"Okay, that does it," the doctor said with mock severity. "We're trading places." He put his stethoscope around Jobi's neck. As she wiggled in delight, he put the earpieces in her ears and placed the other end on his own chest.

"What do you hear?" he asked anxiously.

"The Monkeys—and they've got a good beat." With this Jobi exploded into peals of laughter. I joined her, and Dr. McMillan stood grinning, shaking his head in amusement.

He proceeded to examine her, joking and chatting with her all the while. He managed to get in a few real questions, which I realized were designed to see if she was healing emotionally as well as physically.

"She looks great," he smiled at me. Then, turning to Jobi, "For a rather squirrelly person."

The doctor handed me a slip of paper and told me to take her up to the X-ray section for chest films. He patted my shoulder and promised they'd call the next day with the results.

The taking of chest X rays is, of course, a relatively simple and painless procedure for any patient. It's the mother and father of the patient who suffer the pain of waiting for results. As requested, I carried the developed pictures back down to pediatrics to leave them with Dr. McMillan's nurse. Halfway down a corridor, feeling like a spy, I removed an X ray from its envelope.

I recognized ribs and a neck and two baglike things I assumed were lungs. I studied the picture, once imagining I saw a hideous little spot in one lung. It was a fingerprint. I realized I wouldn't recognize a real spot if I, God forbid, saw one. Sighing, I put the X ray back in the envelope. I would just have to wait until the next day.

I'm not a good waiter. I glued myself to the phone the next day, wishing I were a nail biter. David kept calling me to find out if I had heard any news. So did my mother, my grandmother, two aunts, and an uncle.

At three o'clock that afternoon, I was through waiting. I called the clinic. The line was busy. How can a medical clinic's line be busy? What if someone was dying? No—dumb thought.

I dialed again. This time a voice answered. "Suburban Medical Clinic. Will you hold, please?"

I was about to answer, "No way!" when she clicked off, leaving me in that helpless silence that meant I was on hold. I considered hanging up three times in the ten minutes she left me "holding." But what good would that do? I'd just have to repeat the whole frustrating process.

Finally, the voice returned. "May I help you?"

"Yes—I want to speak to Dr. McMillan or his nur . . ."

"Hold, please." She left me again. I vowed if I ever found out who she was, her days would be numbered.

Five minutes passed. A new voice. "Pediatrics. Sally speaking."

"I'd like to speak to Dr. McMillan, please." Rather polite, considering my mood.

"Just a moment, please." I've heard that one before.

I waited four more minutes in the familiar void of hold. I wondered, Am I actually going to speak to Dr. McMillan? Don't be silly.

"This is Jane. May I help you?" It could be worse. Jane is Dr. McMillan's nurse.

"Jane, this is Sharon Halper. Do you have the results of Jobi's X rays?"

"Just a minute, Mrs. Halper, I'll check."

Barely controlling an urge to cry "Wait! Please . . . don't leave me," I managed a civil "All right."

She came back a few minutes later. "Mrs. Halper? The X rays are fine."

"Thank you." You couldn't have called me hours ago and told me that, could you? Instead you made me go sleepless through the night, allowed me to nearly die with worry all day, and left me on hold for nearly a half hour.

But I didn't say all that. I still hadn't learned.

18

"I THINK WE SHOULD GET ANOTHER OPINION."

David still had said nothing to me about his research. He had collected an incredible amount of medical data for a layman. There were fifteen or twenty file cards held in a neat pile by a rubber band. He kept them in his briefcase. The cards bore the names of doctors, medical centers, and nearly unpronounceable drugs.

Later I would look at one card, which had a single word printed neatly in the center: Adriamycin. The drug had been mentioned by three doctors—but they said it was unavailable. Something about a strike at the factory where it was made in Italy. Imagine children dying because of a strike. No, don't.

"Another opinion about what?" I asked. We had just turned off the television in our bedroom after watching the ten o'clock news. I opened a novel and propped the pillows more firmly behind me.

"You know about what," David said wearily. He knew he was on dangerous ground, but he needed more ammunition to fight my continuing passive attitude. He even knew from where the second opinion was to come.

Like most Twin City residents, David still felt deeply rooted respect and a kind of awe for the University of Minnesota Hospital. People were flown to University Hospital from all over the world for specialized treatment. Its reputation and mystique were topped only by that of the Mayo Clinic, but the university medical facility ran a close second in David's estimation.

66

During his research, David had learned of Dr. Scott Nelson, who was chief of pediatric oncology at the university. The doctor enjoyed a reputation for skilled medicine and liberal ideas. He had sounded like just the person David needed.

"Sweetheart," David pulled me over to him in the bed. "Come on," he pleaded as I stiffened. "I just think we owe it to Jobi to get one more opinion."

I relaxed and laid my head on his shoulder. "Another doctor. Another examination. More bad news."

"I know how you feel. And I know how much you like Dr. McMillan. But I'll bet he'd agree with me." David had never met Dr. McMillan, but he was grasping at straws.

"Well," I sighed. "Dr. McMillan did offer to bring in someone else the first time I met him."

"All right then," David jumped on my first sign of surrender. "Even Dr. McMillan knows the value of a consultation. I heard about someone at University Hospital—a Dr. Nelson. He's the head of pediatric oncology over there, and he's supposed to be tops."

"Where did you hear about him?" I moved away again.

"From my Uncle Jerry," David said, obviously hoping I wouldn't question him further. But he needn't have worried.

"That Jerry." I laughed a little with admiration. "He knows everyone in the world."

"Yeah . . . well?"

"Well what?" I asked innocently, turning a page I hadn't even read yet.

"Okay. Quit playing games."

I closed the book and looked at David. He shut his eyes against the tears filling mine.

"If you think it's the right thing to do, David, then okay."

19

WE FOUND OUR WAY through the tangled maze that was the University of Minnesota. Months later, David told me of the memories that besieged him as we drove through the campus.

This was where we had met; where it had all started.

Autumn. Crisp, clear air—tangy with crushed leaves. The campus was electric with Homecoming. Crazy signs decorated the fraternity and sorority houses. "Number One in 1960!"

David felt good. Good—hell! David felt great! He maneuvered his '55 black Chevy convertible through the crush of traffic on University Avenue. He admired the shining hood. He had spent the morning washing and waxing it for that moment. Maroon and gold ribbons were tied to the radio antenna. Students in other cars called out to each other. When a car displayed rival colors, the sound of catcalls and horns blasting filled the street.

David put his arm around the strawberry blonde next to him. My freckled nose wrinkled cutely at him, and I gave a wiggle of excitement. In the backseat, his sister Diane and her boyfriend sang the "Minnesota Rouser" at the top of their lungs.

I looked up at him with large, sparkling blue eyes. "God —I love Homecoming." I planted a kiss on his cheek. David grinned and wondered if he could drop his hand a little lower than my shoulder.

"It doesn't look the same somehow, does it?" I asked, remembering the same things. David drove the 1971 Ford station wagon slowly down the street.

"No. Nothing's the same," he responded quietly.

"Sunshine, this is where Dad and I went to school. We must have driven down this street together a million times."

"I know," Jobi giggled. "And you skipped classes and hid out in the Hillel House so you could be together."

"Fine things you teach your daughter," David accused good humoredly. He dropped his tone suggestively. "Did you tell her about the library on the second floor?"

I turned red and quickly said, "Look, Jobi, there's the Varsity Restaurant. We ate there almost every morning."

David dropped us off at the entrance to the hospital and went to park the car. At the time, I didn't realize how important our visit with Dr. Nelson seemed to him. He felt that the doctor just had to back him up. Everything depended on it.

Two hours later David and I were seated in Scott Nelson's office. Jobi had been left in the waiting room with some children's storybooks.

Dr. Nelson was a pleasant, youngish-looking man with an easy manner. He had known all about Jobi before we arrived. He explained that almost every oncologist in the city knew about her as well as several around the country. Osteogenic sarcoma was so rare, the case would be discussed in many places.

"What conclusions have you drawn, doctor?" I didn't know that David's palms were sweating and he was praying for the right answer.

"Frankly, Mr. Halper, I concur with Dr. McMillan. If it were my patient, I'd do nothing at this time."

I could see David stiffen with anger. "Just do nothing," he repeated the doctor's words bitterly.

"Until such time as treatment becomes necessary because

the tumor recurs," continued Dr. Nelson. He looked at us with compassion. "I know you want me to be honest with you."

David and I nodded—David with tight, compressed lips; I, slowly and sadly, but with relief.

"We've tried every method we know to prevent this disease from returning in other patients. Nothing has ever worked. That's why I counsel you to wait. If and when the malignancy returns, then we'll treat it as aggressively as we can."

"All right." David spat out the words. "And 'if and when' it returns, what is the true likelihood of saving her?"

Scott Nelson looked him directly in the eye and shook his head.

Before we could respond, he said quickly, "But maybe something new will come up by then. We make progress every day."

I wiped my eyes with a tissue and rose to leave. But David wasn't quite finished.

"Doctor, what's your opinion of methotrexate?"

Dr. Nelson looked at him in surprise, but answered readily. "We haven't seen any noticeable results with it."

"Cytoxan, vincristine." David spattered drug names like bullets from a machine gun. Dr. Nelson kept shaking his head.

"Mr. Halper, none of those drugs are any worse or any better than anything else."

"What about Adriamycin?"

"Adriamycin—how did you hear about that?"

"Is it effective?" David persisted.

"Not in my opinion. It's brand new. Besides, no one can get it. There's a . . ."

"I know," David broke in. "There's a strike in Italy."

Dr. Nelson held up his hands in surrender to David's obvious store of information. He was silent a moment, then,

70

"Look, Mr. Halper . . . Mrs. Halper . . . the fact of the matter is no one has an answer for you. Lots of people may tell you many different things. Your own judgment is probably as good as anyone else's at this point. Eventually it all boils down to your personal philosophy of life."

Nelson softened his tone and added gently, "I'm only telling you if it were my little girl—I wouldn't use any treatment."

"Thank you for your time, Dr. Nelson," David said crisply and ushered me quickly from the office. I had been staring openmouthed at him while he name-dropped drugs. He probably expected a tirade of questions from me. But my mind was in turmoil and I said nothing . . . then.

20

I BANGED CUPBOARD DOORS angrily as I prepared dinner that night. Where had David come up with those drug names he used in Dr. Nelson's office? The alien words had rolled glibly off his tongue. Why? What had he been doing behind my back? David knew how I felt about using drugs on Jobi.

But it was all right. Dr. Nelson had fixed David's wagon. He was the third doctor to agree it was best to leave Jobi alone. I remembered the day Dr. Parrish and I had coffee together at the hospital.

I had related the highlights of my first meeting with Dr. McMillan, and Josephine Parrish had nodded approvingly.

"I'm glad to hear Dr. McMillan isn't in favor of treatment. It's the way I feel too."

I smiled gratefully. "I kind of thought you'd agree."

Dr. Parrish covered my hand with her own. "The thing I've been hoping is that you wouldn't become a runner."

"What do you mean, a runner?"

Dr. Parrish paused a moment. "So many people in your situation run from one medical source to another—spending all the money they have, exhausting themselves, and living on false hopes—all for nothing."

"No," I had said firmly. "Not us."

Now here was David spouting horrible-sounding drugs like so many dirty words. Well, we'd have it out later. Nobody, I thought fiercely, is going to cause that child to suffer again.

The child in question could be heard giggling in the family room. Judy Sher and another neighbor child, Sue Brennon, had come to visit, and they were playing happily at one of their favorite games—operation. I had the shudders the first time I heard them play the game. It seemed macabre to me. But it held great fascination for the children, and they took turns being doctor, nurse, and patient. When Jobi was the doctor, she always had to amputate something —even an ear once—and the girls would laugh and act silly as only eight-year-olds can.

"I'm sorry, madam, but we're going to have to take off your elbow today and maybe your right baby toe."

"Oh, no, doctor. I need those things."

"That's the way it goes."

That day their mock drama annoyed me more than usual. I supposed it was just spillover from the meeting with Dr. Nelson that afternoon, and I controlled my urge to tell the girls to go home.

Dinner was tense and the children reacted by squabbling with each other. David's nerves must have been as taut as mine, because he finally lost his temper and sent Heidi to her room.

"Oh sure," she cried over her shoulder. "It's always me. Never Jobi. Well I hate Jobi!"

No one had any appetite after that, so dinner ended. When David and I finally got into bed that night, I was close to tears. But I steeled myself and turned to him.

"Where did you get the names of all those drugs?"

He sighed. "Why did you wait so long to ask? I've been waiting all day."

"Well I surely wasn't going to discuss it in front of Jobi," I snapped.

"Okay . . ." He plunged in. "I've been speaking to medical centers all over the country."

"But why, David? Why?"

"Because I cannot sit here and wait for Jobi to die. That's why," he shouted at me. I burst into tears, his words tearing into me like a knife.

"I'm sorry—I'm sorry," he pleaded, taking me in his arms. "I shouldn't have said that. It's just that I'm so damned frustrated."

"I know," I murmured, trying to stop crying. "How do you think I feel? Do you think I want her to . . . to . . ." and a fresh wave of sobbing overtook me.

"Listen to me," David ordered, shaking me gently. "There are people out there who have different answers than the ones we've been getting—better answers."

"Like who?" I asked, blowing my nose. "Who are these people you're talking about?"

"I have it all written down on file cards; the names of doctors prominent in cancer research, famous medical centers, and yes, new drugs."

"And I'll bet you have them all filed in order according to how poisonous they are," I said bitterly.

"Will you stop throwing up smoke screens and listen to me?" He raised his voice again. "I've been at this for weeks. I've got a lot of valuable information.

73

"Sharon, sweetheart, we've got to give her a chance. We'll never forgive ourselves if we don't even try. We'll wonder the rest of our lives if we could have saved her and didn't."

We both lay back on the pillows. Tears still trickled down my cheeks, and David's eyes were red and watery.

I reached for his hand. "Will you let me think about it?"

"Of course," he breathed, drawing me close. "That's all I'm asking you to do."

We held each other for a while, and then David fell asleep. But that relief was denied me. Finally, I got up quietly and put on my robe. I made my way down the steps without turning on a light and sat in the kitchen. The room was faintly illuminated by reflections from the snow through the patio doors. I looked out and little pictures flickered across the ghostly yard.

In the apple tree, Jobi danced with the Park Petites—a junior dance team that performed at a Viking game one summer. How funny she looked in that pink satin derby. It was so large, it kept falling down on her nose.

And there, in the rock garden, Jobi wore her long pink formal. There was a flower wreath in her shining hair. She was a finalist in the St. Louis Park Junior Queen pageant. She looked like an angel in the parade, riding the float like topping on a cake.

Jobi.

I went up the stairs and entered her room. She was fast asleep, the portable intercom we had installed humming slightly. I had been worried she would need me some night and I wouldn't hear her. The intercom made me feel better. Except for the times she moaned and keened with phantom pains in her sleep.

But she was quiet now. I looked down at the delicate sleeping figure. Suddenly, she was gone. Only a faint gold haze marked the place her body had been.

Overpowering, overwhelming loneliness filled me. I was

suffocating with loss. My eardrums throbbed with the emptiness of the bed . . . the emptiness of the room.

"No," I moaned softly. "Please, no . . ."

I blinked the searing tears from my eyes and reached out to touch the empty pillow. My fingers slid across smooth soft skin, warm and slightly damp with sleep. They buried themselves in silky hair and pulled the covers over flannel-clad shoulders. I kissed the soft temple, a tiny butterfly pulse beating beneath it.

I went back into our bedroom and crept into bed. I lay as close to David's sleeping warmth as I could. I slept.

21

DAVID PARKED THE MAROON station wagon in front of the semidarkened medical center. The night was very dark, and cold mist seemed to envelop us as we walked to the entrance.

He held my elbow so I wouldn't fall on one of the icy patches dotting the parking lot. I knew he could feel my trembling through my coat. The light over the door splashed eerily onto our faces.

Now I led the way down the carpeted hallway to Dr. McMillan's office. I had been here before. McMillan and Dr. Parrish were waiting. Josephine Parrish sat tensely in a straight-back chair. The other doctor lounged calmly against his desk.

"David, this is Dr. McMillan. Doctor, my husband, David." My voice shook slightly and sounded brittle in my own ears.

The two men shook hands and sized each other up. Dr. McMillan's smile remained on his lips, but faded from his eyes. David didn't even bother to smile.

He looked at Charles McMillan . . . the suntanned handsome face. I could almost hear my husband thinking, "Probably took a vacation on my money." David took in the distinguished-looking gray hair and faintly amused expression in the doctor's ice blue eyes. Again I sensed his thoughts, "Cocky bastard."

David had admitted to me that he started to dislike the man the moment I had begun extolling his virtues. In David's opinion, McMillan's passive attitude had set back by weeks his campaign to get Jobi on treatment.

This first meeting between the two men did nothing to promote better feelings.

Dr. McMillan sat on the edge of his desk, folded his arms, and raised one eyebrow. "Would you like to sit down, Mr. Halper?" McMillan asked politely.

"I'd prefer to stand." The combatants had squared off.

The meeting had been arranged by Josephine Parrish. When, to David's intense relief, I had relented and agreed Jobi should be given treatment, he sat me down in the kitchen and literally layed his cards on the table.

"You called all these places?" I was incredulous.

"And others. I only kept records of the places that sounded promising."

"I can't read them," I said softly. David chose to believe I meant his handwriting was bad.

"Bethesda. High-dose methotrexate," he read.

"What's that?"

"A type of chemotherapy. They give a toxic dose of the drug, then later, some kind of antidote—they call it a rescue."

"Forget that one. It's horrible-sounding."

76

"Hey—none of them want to give her sugar pills," he said gently.

"I know. But—David, that sounds like poison," I pleaded.

"All right. Forget Bethesda."

We reviewed the rest of the cards. There was nothing to guide our decision but instinct.

"When I spoke to these people, I started to feel as though each one was an octopus and was reaching out tentacles to try and get her," David had said as we sipped hot tea, resting from our study.

"I suppose she's a real choice morsel," I remarked dryly. "They don't get too many like Jobi to play with."

Houston was the final choice. More than a place—a name —Jordan Wilbur. Dr. Wilbur had developed a fine reputation for pioneering work with children suffering from all kinds of cancer. When we learned he was at present doing a protocol study involving several other children with osteogenic sarcoma, there was nothing more to discuss.

"He's the man to put Jobi on chemotherapy," David decided positively.

"Maybe we should talk to this Dr. Wilbur and hear what he has to say," I said hesitantly.

Dr. Parrish had been called upon to arrange a meeting between us, Dr. McMillan, and herself at a time convenient to the two doctors. McMillan would have to make the actual arrangements for Jobi's appointment with Jordan Wilbur and take care of any follow-up work. Dr. McMillan had agreed to the meeting, but not to the plan.

"Frankly, I have to tell you folks that I spoke to Scott Nelson at the U., and I have to go along with his thinking," said Dr. McMillan firmly.

David said coldly, "That's all well and good, but we've already made our decision. We're taking Jobi to Wilbur in Houston and putting her on chemotherapy."

77

"Well," I said timidly. "We're going to talk to him about it."

I was ignored.

McMillan straightened and said tightly, "Mr. Halper, anything that can be done, could be done right here."

"Really, doctor? Can you get Adriamycin?" Everyone in the room knew that he couldn't. Dr. McMillan's face became livid. David felt the heat in his own face as he pushed harder. "Dr. Wilbur can get Adriamycin. In fact he's the only one in the country who has it, doctor."

"That may be, Mr. Halper. But I don't agree that Adriamycin will make any difference."

The room was electric. Dr. Parrish and I watched helplessly as David took a step closer to Dr. McMillan. His eyes narrowed. His fists clenched unconsciously.

"Dr. McMillan." Now his words were like bee stings. "I don't care whether you agree or disagree. I'm not even interested in your opinion."

"David . . ." I rose to try and halt David's bitter flow of words. But he was lost in anger and scarcely heard me. All he could see was this man standing in the way of his attempt to save Jobi's life.

"What I need you for," David continued through clenched teeth, "is to make the arrangements. Period."

The muscles in Charles McMillan's jaw moved. Anger glittered from his eyes. The skin around his lips was white. David tensed. I knew he wanted to punch the man and he hoped McMillan would make a move.

"All right—just hold everything." Josephine Parrish stepped between the two men. "Chuck, I feel like you, that this trip to Houston isn't necessary. But on the other hand, if that's what they want, we have to help them do it."

David and Dr. McMillan stared at her for a moment. Then McMillan looked at my face, tears rolling down my

78

cheeks. He smiled slightly. "All right. If that's the way they want it."

David let his breath out slowly and unclenched his fist.

We prepared to leave. Dr. Parrish and I walked ahead, discussing Jobi. As David started through the door, Dr. McMillan gave a parting thrust.

"Mr. Halper . . . you're not going to Houston."

David whirled, about to explode.

McMillan chuckled at his expression. "Wilbur moved his whole operation to San Francisco . . . Palo Alto, to be exact."

22

A WHEELCHAIR did amazing things in Disneyland. It dissolved long Christmas vacation lines in front of rides. And no one got mad. It wiped the mechanical expression off the faces of ticket takers and replaced it with soft smiles. And it drew the stares of strangers.

Everyone looked at the little girl with long burnished pigtails and a smile that seemed too wide for her face. Everyone looked at her pinned-up pant leg.

But Jobi didn't care. She looked at the wonder of Walt Disney's creation and decided she must be in heaven. Her little brother Jonathan's eyes had been big brown circles of astonishment, perhaps even a little fear, since the family had arrived in California. He stayed close to his father, holding on to his jacket most of the time. Heidi was flushed with excitement and kept adding to the list of rides she wanted to take.

Even David was infected by the magic of Disneyland. He

didn't complain about the money we were spending even once.

As we rode the little cars through Small World, the most enchanting ride I've ever been on, I hugged Jobi to me and looked at the pleasure in the faces of my family. I was so glad we had come.

The trip had almost been canceled when Jobi's phantom pains grew so intense, she woke us several times each night.

"How can we take her on a trip?" David had asked almost angrily one night a few days before we were scheduled to leave. She had been crying most of the night, each moan and sob filtering through the intercom on my nightstand.

"It won't be easy," I said wearily, getting out of bed for the fourth time that night. Not that I had much comfort to give her, but how could I sleep when she suffered so?

"Maybe we should go right to San Francisco and forget Disneyland and Hawaii," David said, rolling on his back and staring at the ceiling in the dusky light of five in the morning.

"But we promised," I protested. "Not just Jobi—you can't do that to the other kids."

"Just think what it's going to be like," he said quietly.

"No. I don't want to think about it. I just want to do it."

We argued again a few times, but in the end, we went.

Two days in Disneyland were fun, exciting, and more than enough. On the evening of the second night, we settled three sleepy bundles on a big 747 bound for Hawaii. The three appeared to be children, but in reality were sacks full of hot dogs, ice cream, and popcorn smeared liberally with cotton candy and shaken well on nearly every ride at Disneyland. I hoped fervently all three bundles would keep their contents on the inside during the flight. But I had a few doubts.

We arrived in the Hawaiian airport at midnight on Christmas Eve. I'd like to report we were greeted by grass-skirted dancers bearing flower leis, but I can't. We weren't even greeted by the limousine we had prepaid for before we left home. The airport was deserted.

We stood in the middle of the silent airport. Was everyone else at home roasting chestnuts in an open fire, or maybe roasting a pig at a luau? I wasn't sure what people did in Hawaii on Christmas Eve.

Jobi sat languidly in her wheelchair, the pink crutches across her lap but dragging on the floor. Jon dozed on his father's shoulder, and Heidi drooped sleepily. David looked at me helplessly.

"Aloha," I said.

We finally found a cab driver who appeared to think it was our fault he had to work on Christmas. David's tip reflected his refusal to accept the blame.

We stayed in Hawaii for ten days, and it never got any better.

We woke up each morning. Got everybody dressed. Went down to the Rigger, a fairly inexpensive restaurant we found, for breakfast. Jobi wouldn't eat. Heidi ordered more than she could eat, and David yelled. Jon wanted Froot Loops—they didn't have Froot Loops. Everyone stared at Jobi.

Back up to our room. Got everybody into bathing suits. Down to the beach. Found mats—found space. "Don't go too deep, Heidi." "Jonathan, quit throwing sand on that lady." "David, Jobi wants to go in the water." "Wait, I'll unwrap her Ace bandage." Everyone stared at Jobi.

Lunch time. Put on cover-ups and trooped across the street to McDonald's. I couldn't look at a McDonald's again, but I said nothing. The magic of Disneyland was gone, and David had started complaining about money again. I tried a fish sandwich. I thought there was sand in it. No one was staring at Jobi because a man came into the restaurant wearing a dress and high heels.

After lunch we showered and changed everyone. It took only two hours. There was sand all over the bedroom and

81

an inch deep in the bathtub. We were going on a tour. The sights were beautiful, and the children would rather have been at the beach. Heidi got car sick in the bus. Everyone stared at Jobi.

Dinner—we would try something nice tonight. A special treat. Very expensive, but David couldn't look at another McDonald's either. Jobi wouldn't eat. Heidi ordered more than she could eat, and David yelled. Jon wanted a McDonald's burger. We walked back to the hotel because the night was so lovely. A couple walked past us staring and whispering. They turned back and the woman said, "What happened to your little girl? Was she in a car accident?" David smiled nastily and said, "No. It's a football injury." The couple hurried away.

Wall-to-wall children in our room at night. Lovemaking? We were lucky still to be speaking to each other by the end of the day. Oh well. At least Jobi's phantom pains were gone. Maybe they didn't like Hawaii either.

Only one bright spot marked that miserable ten days in paradise. A group of Japanese students befriended us on the beach. Hawaii was filled with Japanese tourists while we were there. David later told our friends there were "ten thousand Japanese with thirty thousand cameras."

They were very polite people; the only ones who didn't stare at Jobi. David thought it was because they had seen so much of the same thing in their own country after Hiroshima. It was a sobering thought.

The students we met were teenagers, perhaps fifteen or sixteen. They always smiled and giggled when we looked their way, and I had assumed they spoke no English.

But one day, a pretty young girl in the group came over and sat on our blanket, smiling and giggling more enthusiastically than usual.

"For you," she said shyly, and gave Jobi a little Japanese toy. With broken English, smiles, and gestures, she explained it was a game and taught the children how to play it. The rest of her friends came over to see how the game was progressing, and soon everyone was laughing and teaching each other new words.

"O-hi-o," said five-year-old Jonathan the next morning, bowing formally.

"Sayonara," I replied, sending him back to bed. It was six o'clock.

PART TWO

23

JOBI DIDN'T KNOW ABOUT Palo Alto and Dr. Wilbur. And chemotherapy. I couldn't bear to spoil her fun in Disneyland and Hawaii. All three children thought we were stopping in San Francisco on our way home to visit my cousin Paul.

Paul. Destroyer of his parents' hopes and dreams; creator of mine.

We were sitting on the floor of his tiny, ancient apartment in a shabby section of San Francisco. Paul's gentle wife, Cindy, served us fruit and nuts and herb tea. She reminded me of a doe, with her slender body and graceful movements.

Paul smiled and offered me a fig imported from some exotic-sounding place. His eyes locked into mine, and I saw he was no longer the boy I had grown up with. Who was he now?

I knew who he had been. Everyone did. He was Paul Katzovitz—tall, strong, incredibly handsome. He was so popular, the fraternities fought over him, and so did the co-eds. He was brilliant in school, showed great promise as a musician, possessed impeccable manners and *davened*, prayed, with his father in *shul*, synagogue, on Saturday mornings. Paul had been the pride of his parents; the envy of parents whose children were only ordinary.

Until he broke their hearts.

He was graduated with honors from law school in Chicago, passed the bar, and was immediately accepted into the district attorney's office. What a triumph. He married a nice

87

Jewish girl from a good family, of course, and everyone lived happily ever after. For a year.

Then one day, Paul sold his and Cindy's twenty thousand dollars' worth of wedding gifts for a few hundred dollars. He bought a pair of jeans and a backpack for each of them. They closed the door of their chic glass and chrome apartment, left their designer clothes in the closet, and began hitchhiking westward.

Paul's carefully styled curly brown hair began to grow halfway down his back. He pulled it away from his face with a shoelace when it bothered him. But the wild, unkempt beard that appeared during the trip was allowed to blow in the wind.

Cindy, spoiled, pampered child of indulgent upper-middle-class parents, stopped wearing makeup, and when she and her husband ran short of money, she cleaned other people's houses.

Why did they do it? It was a shame, a tragedy—and definitely a mystery. My Uncle Harvey, proud father, cried when he heard. My Bauby moaned and thanked God Zady wasn't alive to know. The rest of the family, those parents of ordinary children, in deep secret places within themselves, didn't feel as badly as they claimed.

"What do you do, Paul?" asked David. That's what gentlemen always ask each other.

"I meditate," Paul answered serenely.

David choked on the handful of nuts he had tossed into his mouth. Cindy smiled sweetly and poured him some more herb tea.

"For a living?" David didn't mean to sound sarcastic. Yes, he probably did.

Paul shrugged. "If we need something, I tune pianos and Cindy cleans a church twice a week."

I looked unbelievingly at Cindy. The last time I'd seen her, she had a daily maid for her four-room apartment.

"What else do you do?" I asked.

Paul looked at me, and his face softened. Warmth seemed to radiate from him. "We simply . . . are."

Cindy and Paul exchanged a gaze. She placed her hand on his arm for a moment. They turned the smile they had given to each other toward us, and it was so sweet, it almost hurt.

Cindy jumped up and said, "Who wants to help crush leaves for more tea?"

The children all clamored to be the one, and Cindy said she had jobs for each of them. They followed her to the small old-fashioned kitchen.

David and I stayed with Paul. No one spoke for a while. I had the feeling Cindy took the children out by prearranged plan.

I looked around the shabby room and then back at Paul. He pushed a long, unruly strand of hair behind his ear. I had known him all my life, but even his eyes were unfamiliar to me. They shone with some inner force, almost fanatical, yet full of peace.

"Why, Paul?" I asked.

He smiled with painful sweetness again. "I found something. I always knew it was somewhere, and I went to look. It's here."

"Here in this apartment?" David scoffed incredulously, gesturing toward the dingy, almost bare room.

"Here—where I am," said Paul simply.

"And where is that, Paul?" I asked gently. Somehow I had the feeling it was important for me to know.

"A place of peace and enlightenment. A place for the mind to live and grow and reach out to help others get here too."

He spoke with such depth and warmth, the intensity of his words wrapped around me. But David's face still wore its cynical look.

"And I suppose all this peace comes from meditation and eating fruit and nuts." David indicated the table we had been served lunch from.

"Yes, that. We're vegetarians now. We eat the things that will bring health to our bodies, and we meditate to bring health to our minds. But there's more."

The sincerity of Paul's feelings began to affect even David. He stopped munching nuts and looking bored. He even leaned forward a little in expectation.

"When I heard you were coming here with Jobi, I suddenly felt very excited. I knew there was an extra purpose to my life." Paul's face was flooded with joy, his eyes damp with emotion. "There's someone I'd like you to meet. His name is Eldon Gunderson, and he can help you."

I looked at him intently. "Help us . . . you mean with Jobi?"

Paul smiled deeply. "With Jobi—with all of you—with all things."

He was about to lose David again. "Hey, if you're talking about some kind of religious nut or faith healer . . ."

"No. Nothing like that," Paul reassured him. "Eldon is a medium. A spirit named Wang, who lived two thousand years ago, speaks through him."

I looked at Paul in astonishment. Was he serious? I glanced at David, hoping he wouldn't laugh in Paul's face. I had done some research into ESP and related phenomena for a term paper and still felt open-minded about such things. But David was a confirmed skeptic.

"Right, Paul," David snorted derisively. "And I suppose this spirit is going to cure Jobi. Come off it."

Paul was undisturbed. He asked gently, "Have either of you heard of Edgar Cayce?"

I knew of the man, David gave a curt, "No."

"Edgar Cayce was a man who could diagnose the cause of illness without seeing a patient," Paul explained. "He was an incredible man. There are hundreds of documented cases involving his powers."

"What do you mean, he diagnosed the cause of illness?

90

Was he a doctor?" David's voice was still heavy with sarcasm. But I could tell he was interested, in spite of himself.

"I read about him," I commented. "He wasn't a doctor, but he appeared to have ESP or something like that."

"It was more than just that," Paul continued. "Cayce would go into a trance and, given the name, location, and symptoms of a sick person, describe exactly what was wrong in medical terms. Later, he couldn't even remember the words he'd used while in the trance."

"That's a fact, David," I added. "There's been a lot of books written about the man."

"Okay—so what's all this got to do with your two-thousand-year-old spirit?"

Paul looked directly at David before answering. Calmly, he ignored the challenge in David's eyes. "Through Eldon Gunderson, Wang can diagnose disease and help us learn all we need to know about ourselves."

Paul paused for a moment, but when David didn't give the expected negative response, he added, "I have arranged for you to meet with Eldon tonight."

David looked as though he were going to object. "I want to go see him, David," I said quickly. From the depth of my fear, I would leave no road to hope untraveled.

"Okay, Paul," said David with a knowing smirk. "How much is this little meeting going to cost me?"

"There's no charge, David." Paul's eyes twinkled a little with amusement. He knew David well enough to realize his last statement had just clinched the deal.

24

THEY WERE ORDINARY-LOOKING people, really. Eldon Gunderson was of medium build with brown hair and warm eyes. He was an accountant, or had been before the spirit of Wang requested him for host. Cara, his wife, was tall and slender, possessed of a gentle smile and soft voice.

Their two children, an elfin girl of ten and a wiry twelve-year-old boy, led Heidi, Jonathan, and Jobi to a room in the rear of the old, but spacious apartment. They could be heard making the happy sounds of new friendship as we were ushered into the living room.

Paul and Cindy flopped on the patterned area rug with familiarity. There were large, comfortable-looking pillows scattered about. These and a plumply upholstered chair were the only furniture, but there were many lit candles about, and the room was friendly.

Cara said we should make ourselves comfortable, which obviously meant to sit on the floor. I sat cross-legged, my back straight—a position I often assumed. Strangely, a memory of my grandfather sitting in that exact manner drifted across my mind. David was anything but relaxed and kept shifting around nervously.

Eldon sat in the armchair facing us, and Cara leaned against a pillow near him on the floor. The flickering candles made shadows and light dance across our upturned faces, as everyone looked at Eldon expectantly.

I was filled with a peculiar excitement, even a little fear. I told myself this was just for fun; an evening's entertainment.

Nothing serious, of course. But my pulse quickened as I watched the man in the armchair compose himself.

He let his hands rest lightly on his thighs and looked past our heads. His features relaxed and his mouth sagged slightly. His eyelids fluttered and he tilted his head back for a moment. Then he opened his eyes and looked at us, his expression serene and kind.

"This man and this woman have a man-child and two female children," said Eldon Gunderson. But it didn't sound like Eldon Gunderson anymore. The voice was ancient and infinite. Open-minded, even a touch skeptical, at that moment I felt I was in an alien presence. The hairs on my arms prickled.

The voice of Wang continued. Eldon's body was totally immobile; only his lips moved. "This man and this woman have love but no happiness between them. The first female child cleaves to the woman, the man-child is of the man. The second female child, that one known as Sun, is a spirit hovering over all. Peace."

After the word peace, the man closed his eyes and bowed his head. I had given a slight gasp when he said "Sun." There was no way he could have known that pet name. Even if my cousin had been inclined to give him information about us in advance, Paul had been away from home too long to have been aware we called Jobi Sunshine.

Cara ignored my expression of surprise and explained, "When Wang says, 'Peace,' he is finished with a statement and invites you to ask a question if you wish."

I tried to catch David's eye, but he was staring intently at Eldon Gunderson; whether in belief or disbelief, I couldn't tell. It was quiet in the room. I was afraid to ask my question, but it was time.

"Will our daughter, Jobi, live?" The question hung in the air like a black shadow. Eldon's eyelids flickered. He shook his head once and, in his own voice, muttered, "Don't understand . . . figures . . . numbers . . . equations. All right."

Then he became still and his eyes opened once more. The voice of Wang filled the room.

"It is not for us to say if the female child lives or dies. A spirit such as hers is only loaned to this earth. How long you may keep her is not known." A pause, some rapid eye movement, then, "This medical facility to which you take the child is fitting. There is a problem with oxygenation of the blood and vitamin deficiencies. This they will find. There is one there in a high place who believes as we. He can help. Peace."

Disappointment and wonder filled me at the same time. I had wished for more, and yet my hopes soared.

More questions and answers took place that night, but the memory of the first exchange between Wang and me is so poignant, so full, it blocks the rest. I knew that even David asked questions of Wang, technical medical questions—probably to test him—and very specific answers were given. But none of that penetrated my mind.

Later, lying next to David in a motel, I listened to the sounds of my children sleeping in cots around us. My thoughts kept returning to the voice of Wang emerging from Eldon Gunderson's lips.

"The first female child cleaves to the woman," he had said. Heidi and me? But she was the most difficult of my children for me to understand. Was it possible her independent, rebellious nature was only a facade? Did she really have a need to be closer to me? And that business about the man-child being "of the man" was true enough. Jonathan was David's shadow. They even walked alike. Then I smiled into the darkness remembering Wang's description of "the one known as the Sun . . . a spirit hovering over all." It was a beautiful fact that anyone entering Jobi's world was warmed by her love.

Wang, or maybe just Eldon Gunderson, had seen deeply into us. He had even mentioned the love, but lack of happiness in David's and my marriage. Of course, Jobi's illness had

94

prompted a sort of truce between us. And the fight for her life gave us a common bond, a cause that drove our personal problems into a far-off corner. We gave each other what we could, and the rest would have to wait.

The puzzling memory was that of Wang's statement about "one in a high place who believes as we." Someone at Stanford Hospital for Children who believed in spirits? That part was, of course, nonsense. Probably it all was nonsense.

The hospital. We'd be going there tomorrow morning in the rented car, a small yellow Gremlin. Jonny couldn't pronounce Gremlin and called it a "Gremil." The girls laughed at him, but the name stuck. Jobi didn't know it yet, but tomorrow morning Jonny's "Gremil" would take her on a journey to still another kind of world. A world that scared me far more than the world of spirits.

25

I WATCHED UNSEEN as Jobi moved slowly along the corridor in front of the cases. Her eyes were round with wonder at the beautiful dolls enclosed in glass and wood. I knew her fingers tingled with the need to touch the fine cream lace dress of a large doll with delicately painted features. Jobi had never seen clothes like those the dolls wore, although later she told me some of them reminded her of the costumes in my shows. The woman who brought her to the dolls told her they belonged to someone named Shirley Temple. Jobi didn't know who she was, but decided this Shirley Temple was a very lucky little girl.

As Jobi passed a case of miniature dolls in exotic costumes, her image was reflected in the glass. It made her look like a giant hovering omnipotently over a world of tiny people. But in an ankle-length white piqué dress with pink gingham trim, a crisp white bow pulling her long blond hair back from her forehead, the giant looked friendly enough. She noticed her reflection and, balancing on one white patent leather shoe, waved a crutch benevolently at herself. The crutches, originally glossy pink with happy flowers and butterflies were now chipped and beaten, the pattern obscured. The sandy beaches of Hawaii had not been kind to her artwork.

Another ghostly figure moved along the glass, and Jobi turned to watch a child passing by her. The child was a little younger than Jobi—a girl—but this fact was obvious only because the girl wore a faded summer dress and scuffed ankle-strap shoes. There was no other claim to femininity in the small figure, with its birdlike arms and legs, pale face, and hairless skull.

Jobi stared at the child's retreating back. Her face was filled with amazement and pity. "That poor, poor little girl," she told me later. "She didn't have any hair."

She turned back to the doll case, but her interest in them was waning. She was becoming uneasy now, and I knew she was beginning to wonder where I was, and why I was staying away for such a long time. But I needed a few moments to prepare myself.

When we left her to talk to Dr. Wilbur, we said it would be only a few minutes. Now she probably wished she had stayed with Heidi and Jonathan at Paul's house. I could tell she had felt very important when I told her she could come in the "Gremil," but her sister and brother would have to remain behind. Heidi had glared at her and Jobi returned a secret smug smile when she thought I wasn't looking.

Jobi was aware of Heidi's growing dislike for her. Not that the sisters hadn't had plenty of squabbles in the past, but since Jobi's operation, the normal rivalry of a ten-year-old toward her eight-year-old sibling had turned to bitter resentment.

"She doesn't like me 'cause I got all those presents," Jobi had told me. How could I argue in light of Heidi's tight, angry face as day after day, more gifts had arrived. Jobi had given Jonathan some of her books and toys, and he had been perfectly happy. But Heidi refused to be so easily mollified. The tape recorder had caused the final explosion. When the portable tape recorder from David's cousin was delivered to Jobi, Heidi had burst into sobs and run from the room. I shook my head sadly, and went upstairs to try and comfort Heidi, but the nearly hysterical child refused to talk or leave her bedroom.

The next day Heidi said to Jobi, "I don't know why everyone's giving you presents and paying so much attention to you. Just because you don't have a leg. Big deal. Mom said you're going to get a new one pretty soon. So then you'll have the leg *and* the presents." With that Heidi stalked out of the room and had remained distant, even in Disneyland.

Jobi had asked only once about the promised leg. Would it look just like her old one? Would she be able to run on it? Not that it really mattered that much to her. She could swing along faster on her crutches than most of the kids could run. And it seemed as if she could jump rope on her one leg longer and faster than anyone else. Now that it didn't hurt any more, she agreed with Heidi somewhat. Having only one leg was no big deal. Except when people stared. . . .

"Hi, Sunshine." I stepped from behind the case where I had been watching her, and bent to kiss the top of her head.

Jobi smiled in relief to see me at last. "Where's Dad?"

"He had to call his office. You know Dad . . . he's been gone for two weeks, and he thinks everyone stopped buying cartons because he wasn't there."

"That's Dad," Jobi chuckled a little, then she accused me mildly, "You were gone a long time."

97

"Yes." My light tone thickened. "I want to talk to you about what I was doing."

I could sense apprehension filling my child. My lips were still smiling, but not my face. Jobi could tell she wouldn't like what was about to happen. It was the same kind of feeling she told me she had had several months ago . . . right after the boy kicked her leg.

We sat down on a small couch in the airy lobby of the building. I picked up Jobi's hand and held it.

"Jobi, you know you had a tumor, a bad lump, growing in your leg; that's why they had to amputate."

Jobi nodded solemnly. I knew the intuitive little girl could see that I didn't really want to say these words and that I was feeling sad. Jobi stroked my arm comfortingly with her free hand. She didn't like her mother to be sad.

I continued softly. "The doctors in Minneapolis told us the tumor could possibly come back somewhere else in your body. But we heard about a doctor, the tall man you met before, who has some special new medicine that could stop the tumor from ever coming back. That's why we came here. This building is the hospital where Dr. Wilbur takes care of children with . . . problems."

Jobi looked out the window. It was raining. "I saw a girl with no hair."

My voice sounded strange, as though I had swallowed wrong. "The medicines sometimes make people lose their hair. But it always grows back."

"Do the medicines taste icky? I hate icky tastes." Jobi turned back to look at my face.

"Some of them might taste bad, and some of them are shots."

Now Jobi put her hand on her tummy—I knew it was starting to hurt. Her neck grew damp, as it did in the middle of summer.

"Sunshine," I said gently. "You're a little girl, but this is a very grown-up thing we're talking about. I want you to think about this and be part of the decision whether to take the medicines. I won't force you."

Tears began to plop onto Jobi's cheeks.

"Mom . . ."

"Yes, Love."

"I don't think I really have any choice."

I gathered her onto my lap and held her very close. She nestled her wet face against my neck, and our tears mingled. Then I rocked her gently, even though there was no rocking chair.

26

"SHARON . . . IF . . . IF something happens, do you want me to fly back here to bring you home?"

"My God," I said, realizing David meant the possibility of Jobi's death. "Yes—yes, of course."

He was leaving; taking Jonathan and Heidi home. Jobi and I would remain in the Children's Hospital at Stanford. And I was terrified.

Married at eighteen, I had never been away from home unescorted in my life. I had never been on a plane alone or even made a major decision without advice. Since the day of my marriage, I'd never slept anywhere but next to David except when I had babies. Now I was to stay in this strange place for an undetermined amount of time and help the doctors use Jobi as a guinea pig. We were joining a unique society with very exclusive criteria for membership.

Dr. Wilbur had explained how things worked here in his wing at the Children's Hospital.

"Children who have a problem no one else seems able to

solve come to us. The only requirement we have is that each child be accompanied by a family member—a mother, father, aunt, sister—it doesn't really matter. As long as the relative makes a commitment to live here with the child and directly participate in his or her care.

"We feel that personal involvement is as much a part of the treatment as the medical program. Then the child and his or her relative—sometimes entire families move in for a while—become part of the whole community of children and family and staff. We form a circle of hope, love, and protection around each child.

"It's amazing how tightly that circle forms. Everyone helps everyone else and we try to become invincible."

"And are you invincible?" David asked.

"No," Dr. Wilbur replied honestly, if sadly. The fierce determination shone from his intelligent gray eyes. "But we never give up. There's always hope. And our track record is higher than most."

My liking for this dedicated man deepened. I couldn't help but compare him to the gloomy, negative Minneapolis doctors who had all but insisted we should give up on Jobi. Not that Wilbur hadn't explained the risks of his program. He told us point-blank that many children died of complications brought on by the drugs themselves. The program Jobi would be on presented an especially big question mark. It was a protocol study—an experiment—not a cure.

"You know, Dr. Wilbur," I couldn't help saying. "The doctors at home told us only about one out of a hundred children with osteogenic sarcoma live. How much better a chance will the drugs give her?"

"Mrs. Halper, I don't like reducing children to numbers on a piece of paper. Those statistics mean nothing. If one or two or three percent of patients with osteo live, and your daughter is one of those three, you never needed the numbers."

But David was a numbers man through and through. "But what are her chances on chemotherapy?"

Dr. Wilbur smiled tolerantly. "Frankly, the experimental program on this particular disease has been in effect such a short time, we can't state precise chances or odds with any accuracy. But if you must have a number, my educated stab in the dark would be ten percent."

"A ten percent chance for life," I said softly.

"Ten percent is better than one," David spoke firmly. "Even in Vegas."

27

TELLING JOBI ABOUT THE HOSPITAL and drug program was among the saddest moments of my life. Sad, not because she would have to endure the ordeal of chemotherapy, but because when I presented the choice to her, I watched her eyes change from childish innocence to ancient wisdom. I felt that an old soul lived behind those startling green blue eyes with a splotch of brown in one. An old soul who was coming forth to handle what the child could not.

But there was no old soul to help the mother. All through the hideous days and nights when Jobi had her surgery, people continuously remarked to me, "Aren't you a marvel! Aren't you brave! So wonderful how you're bearing up under all this." What did they expect me to do? Swoon and lie under a canopy while my child was operated on? Throw myself on the ground and rend my garment instead of taking care of her? Foolish, lucky people who've known no tragedy.

We all have strength within us to draw upon when there is no choice.

Now I wondered if I had enough reserve left to see me through the next year. I tried to keep the list of risks and dangers out of my mind, as Jobi and I watched David leave with Heidi and Jon. Don't think about white blood cells being destroyed, leaving a child vulnerable to pneumonia, or even death from a simple cold. Forget the possible damage to her heart, her liver, her kidneys. Don't even let your mind approach the future; no one knows what the drugs and constant necessary X rays will do to her female organs. Will they develop? Will she ever have a child?

Jobi waved at the retreating yellow "Gremil." I could see Jonny's face still pressed against the rear window. He had cried and squeezed my legs before he left. He was so young to be without his mother. But it wasn't angry crying. Though we hadn't told any of the children the extreme gravity of Jobi's illness, their instincts were good.

Heidi, pushing jealousy aside for the parting, pressed a small seashell into Jobi's hand. She had found it on the beach in Hawaii, and it was one of her treasures. "Here—you take this," she told her surprised younger sister. "But I want it back when you come home."

Jonathan kissed Jobi shyly and promised generously to play with all her stuffed animals so they wouldn't get lonesome.

"Jon . . ." said Jobi warningly.

"I know," he laughed. "I was kidding."

David hugged me in one of his rare moments of affection. "Don't worry about anything at home. My mother's coming to stay for a while."

I smiled. "David, don't let her run her fingers along the top of the refrigerator looking for dust."

We both laughed, knowing Edythe would do just that. But she would also take very good care of my family for me.

And so they left. My husband and two of my young

children drove away from me in a small yellow car. I didn't know when I'd see them again. Feeling loneliness, fright, and other nameless emotions that threatened to engulf me, I looked down onto Jobi's trusting face. I produced the most cheerful smile I possessed and led Jobi back into the hospital. I squeezed her hand almost as hard as she was squeezing mine.

A year. A year is a lifetime.

This was the first day of the year Jobi would spend as part of an experimental drug program sponsored by the state of California. She would be given a series of cancer-fighting drugs in a three-week sequence. Every three weeks for one year, by injection or pill, Jobi would receive one of the four drugs to be used in her treatment. Cytoxan with vincristine; high-dose methotrexate; Adriamycin. The names seemed to drum in my head like the names of the ten plagues we recite on Passover. Or the names of the concentration camps droned on Yom Kippur. If the cancer didn't get her, the drugs might. But if she beat them both, she would live.

Fighting the depression settling over me like a mantle, I took Jobi back to our room. It was small with one high window, a hospital bed and a cot. There was no bathroom. Along with all the other children and their mothers, we would share the giant bathroom down the hall, complete with stalls, showers, tubs, ironing boards, and supply room. Here were kept linens and towels, which we were free to take as we needed them.

After putting our coats away in the small closet and propping a few of Jobi's toys on her bed, we decided to visit the community kitchen. Ice cream, soda, puddings, and bread for toast were among the food items in one of the two huge refrigerators. The second held personal supplies that were carefully labeled with each child's name. While three meals a day were provided by the hospital, there was a stove in the kitchen for those who wished to prepare their own food. The

103

smell of frying taco shells indicated it was being used as we entered.

Jobi sat on a bench at one of the long tables in the bright, airy room. I found a soda for her and poured myself some coffee from the big pot on a table against the wall. I saw a piece of paper taped to the wall with names on it. There were two Mexican-American women at the stove. One of them noticed me looking at the list and called, "That's who bought coffee. We take turns."

I smiled at her and asked, "Oh—how often does each person buy it?"

She looked at me strangely for a moment and shrugged. Then she turned back to the frying tacos and muttered something in Spanish to her friend. Realization hit me and I felt stupid. How often does a person buy coffee? How often does their child have to come to the hospital? How long will he or she live? I vowed to think before I spoke here in the future. I also made a mental note to buy at least two cans of coffee.

"I think they have ice cream in the freezer. Do you want some?" I asked Jobi, setting down her soda.

She shook her head. "I'm not hungry."

"Hey—you're gonna blow away if you don't start eating." She smiled at me. I was always trying to stuff food into her and stay on a diet myself. It usually worked out the other way around.

A girl in her early twenties entered the kitchen. She was plump, had a long brown ponytail, and wore a green waitress uniform. She was trailed by a small boy of about three. He had the look I had already learned to recognize—white, bloated face and belly; spindly arms and legs; a few stringy wisps of hair clinging to his head—leukemia. The particular drugs used to treat the disease seemed to make all the children look the same. I averted my eyes from the small, sad-looking little boy.

But Jobi was staring at his hand. It was wrapped in

104

gauze and held to a small board with strips of tape. There was obviously a needle in a vein, but it wasn't attached to anything.

"Now Chris, you know I have to go to work. You go watch TV with Mona till supper," the young woman said to the little boy.

"No, Mamma. Don't wanna," the child wailed. "Wanna go wif you."

She noticed Jobi and me sitting at the table and tossed a grin our way before opening the refrigerator. "Hi," she called from inside the freezer section. I could hear her cracking gum loudly. "You must be the new ones."

Chris began to cry louder now, so she raised her voice. "I'm Irene, and the big noise is my son, Chris."

"Happy to meet you," I called back over the steadily rising wail. "My name is Sharon Halper and this is Jo Beth —we call her Jobi."

Irene smiled at Jobi and stuffed half a cherry Popsicle into her son's open mouth. His cries subsided to muffled snuffling and hiccups, as he noisily sucked on the treat. His tears mingled with melting Popsicle and ran onto his white shirt in pink rivulets.

"I'd like to stop and talk, but I'm late for work. Catch you later." Irene exited, her ponytail bobbing and Chris toddling unsteadily after her.

Just then a middle-aged blond woman came into the kitchen and poured herself a cup of coffee. She smiled and sat near us, pushing wispy hair from her forehead.

"Hi. Are you all new here? I'm Emily Denton," she said. But it came out, "Hah—R'y'all new here? Ah'm Em'leh Daynton." She had the heaviest southern drawl I'd ever heard, also the warmest, broadest smile.

"Glad to meet you, Emily." I introduced myself and Jobi.

"Aren't you the prettiest li'l thing ah ever did see," ex-

105

claimed Emily to Jobi, who smiled delightedly. "Too bad you're not a little older. My Robbie'd sure go for y'all."

Before Jobi had a chance to respond to this, Chris could be heard crying with renewed vigor. A nurse hurried past the kitchen in the direction of the sound.

"Irene musta left for work," sighed Emily. "Poor li'l Chris puts up that same howl ever' night."

"Do the nurses take care of him when Irene's gone?" I asked.

"Ever'one takes care o' him. The chile don't have no daddy—ne'er did have one so far as we can tell. Irene has two part-time waitressin' jobs to make ends meet, so we all kinda pitch in and take care o' Chris."

"Is . . . is that little boy going to be all right?" asked Jobi hesitantly.

"They all are, honey," said Emily, patting her hand. "They're all going to be all right." She sipped her coffee and added, almost absently, "Li'l Chris is in a pretty bad way just now, though."

"He has leukemia, doesn't he?" I asked.

"Yes. Leukemia."

There was a clatter and a catcall. A gurney rolled in with a young teenage boy lying facedown on it. He was pushing the wheels himself, his blond hair falling over his thin, but cocky face.

"Hey, Ma!" he yelled. "Where ya been?"

"Hey, biddy buddy. What y'all doin' out here? You're s'posed to be in bed." Emily turned to me. "He had a spinal this mornin' and he i'n't s'posed to move for eighteen hours."

The boy made a sound of disgust. "Ah can't lay there no more. Paula said ah could get around on the gurney if ah keep mah head down."

"Robbie, you'd convince a horned toad to give you his lily pad if you had a mind to. Say hello to Mrs. Halper and Jobi."

"Hi," he said with a decided lack of interest. "Ma—

c'mon. My knees are killin' me. You said you'd get me some ice packs."

"Take it easy, son, ah'm comin'," she said a little more gently. "Y'all go on back to your room and ah'll be along in a minute."

"Well, hurry up." Robbie maneuvered the gurney around and wheeled himself out of the kitchen. Emily sighed wearily and rose. "Honestly, that chile runs me ragged. Listen, he was as rude as a magpie, but his knees are bothersome today and it makes him kinda mean."

"Oh, that's all right," I said quickly. "Please don't apologize."

"When something hurts me, I feel mean too," sympathized Jobi. "What's the matter with his knees?"

"Not to worry, honey. It just some nasty ol' leukemia cells the doctor thinks are collectin' there. But he's got some new medicine they're gonna zap 'im with tomorrow. Then he'll be right again."

Emily pushed her wiry body from the table and cleared her cup. "I'll see y'all later. Hey, Sharon, y'all don't play bridge by any chance."

"I sure do."

She grinned widely and waggled her fingers as she left the room.

28

I CAME TO UNDERSTAND why the stove was a popular item. The dinner provided by the hospital that night consisted of dry, gray roast beef, stiff mashed potatoes with leaden gravy, an unrecognizable vegetable, and sort-of-apple-cobbler.

The meal had come into the kitchen on a huge cart stacked with covered platters—someone had spotted the arrival of the cart and walked up and down the halls of our wing calling, "Soup's on—come and get it."

I brushed Jobi's hair and fluffed up my own curly mop. I was in the grips of a nicotine fit and decided that after dinner I would sneak outside to smoke despite the steady drizzle of rain. I was embarrassed to be a smoker in this place. Probably everyone else had quit in fear, with all the publicity about cigarettes causing cancer. But my need for the ridiculous paper-wrapped leaves overcame a thing so minor as fear.

When Jobi and I entered the kitchen, there were only three or four women and a similar number of children. A very fat Mexican-American boy sat at the table placidly chewing his food. A plump, elderly woman, also Mexican-American, sat across from him anxiously watching his fork travel from his plate to his mouth. When Jobi and I sat near them, she looked up and smiled, her cheeks bulging, eyes crinkling almost closed.

"My grandson, Jose," she indicated the boy, her speech heavily accented. "He is on, *como se dice,* the diet. Mucho fat!" She laughed merrily, her own chubby body billowing. Jobi and I both laughed with her, though Jose didn't break the rhythm of his chewing. He smiled politely around a mouthful.

Emily walked into the room and took a tray off the cart. "Hi, folks," she called to us. "Robbie i'n't feelin' good 'nuf to eat in heah. But meet me later in the smokin' lounge."

Smoking lounge! How could I have missed that when Dr. Wilbur had shown us around the ward? Maybe it was because I didn't notice much else after he had shown us the treatment rooms; tiny cells with heavy doors so the sound of a crying child wouldn't penetrate.

A tall, large-boned man carried a tray to our table. He was accompanied by a girl of about ten with curly brown

108

hair and round brown eyes. She looked at Jobi with interest and said, "Hi. I'm Jo Anna. Who are you?"

Jobi laughed a little and replied, "You're Jo Anna—I'm Jo Beth."

"No kidding," exclaimed the other little girl.

"But I like to be called Jobi best."

"Well, Jobi," boomed Jo Anna's huge companion. "We're happy to meet you." He stuck a huge work-gnarled paw toward Jobi and enclosed her small hand. "Will Painter," he said, next reaching for my hand and pumping it vigorously.

I introduced myself and chatted with Will while the girls made friends. From the corner of my ear I heard Jo Anna speaking rapidly to Jobi. It was strange how solemn the older girl remained. She never smiled as we ate dinner.

From Will Painter I learned that he and his wife, Lee, had two children; a girl of seven and Jo Anna. Lee and their younger daughter would arrive later that evening. The Painters had a camper they used for the six-hour drive to the hospital from their home farther south. One member of the family would sleep in the room with Jo Anna, the other two in the camper parked in the hospital lot. Jo Anna had been a leukemia patient for two years. A recent remission had lasted for six months, causing the Painters' hopes to rise and Jo Anna's hair to grow back. The thick curls she had now didn't even resemble the straight, fine hair she had lost as a result of the drugs. Will said no one seemed to know why the hair grew back differently; just as no one knew why the leukemia cells had suddenly grown active again, or if a new drug, scheduled to be started tomorrow, would have any effect.

Jo Anna asked permission to take Jobi to the game room where they could play Monopoly. Jobi hadn't eaten anything from her tray, but she seemed animated for the first time since we'd arrived, so I agreed.

The two girls left, Jo Anna continuing her steady, unsmiling monologue, Jobi nodding enthusiastically. I noticed

109

that Jo Anna showed no reaction when Jobi pulled her crutches from beneath the table. Will excused himself, and I put the trays back on the cart, determined to find the smoking lounge.

I returned to our small, bare room for my cigarettes, and a sudden surge of fear and loneliness formed a knot in my chest. Self-pity forced me to sit on the edge of Jobi's bed, tears welling up in my eyes. I could never be as brave as Emily with her warm smile, or Will Painter with his hearty handshake, or even the old Mexican-American woman with her fat grandson. Their children were going to die, and they knew it. And yet they behaved as though everything happening here were quite ordinary.

I wanted to go find Jobi and take her away from the hospital. She didn't belong here. This was no place for children—it was Dante's Inferno; where the damned came to pretend.

I knew I was working myself into panic and hysteria. But I couldn't seem to stop the terrible thoughts, tumbling over each other and building until I would scream.

"Phone call for you, Mrs. Halper." The pleasant face of Paula, head nurse, poked into the room. She smiled, ignoring my wet face, and said, "You can get it at the desk."

I nodded and watched her limp away. Paula's right leg was thin and twisted—I recognized a polio victim when I saw one. I followed her to the desk, marveling that she had chosen to be a nurse; all those long hours on her feet—the bending, the lifting. Family, school authorities, everyone had always discouraged me from considering anything but a sitting job with my weak muscles. Where had Paula found the strength? Where had she found the courage?

Paula handed me the phone and turned away behind the desk to give me privacy. "Sharon?" said a familiar voice on the other end of the line. "Are you all right, honey?" It was my mother. I had expected the call to be from Paul or even David, but the sound of that comforting voice brought fresh

110

tears to my eyes. There I stood. A thirty-year-old woman crying because her mother showed up when she was needed.

"Mother—hi—yes, I'm fine. I'm surprised to hear from you so soon." I had spoken to her the day before to let her know our decision to admit Jobi to the hospital.

"Sharon, Dad and I have been discussing this, and we've decided I should come there and stay with you for a while."

"Mother, are you serious?" Shock and wonder filled me. My mother was a white-knuckle flier who had not left her husband's side in thirty-five years.

"Yes, I'm serious. That is, if you want me." There was a hesitation in her voice. If I want her? At that moment I never wanted anything more in my life than to have my mother with me. But I knew what the ordeal of flying and being parted from my father would cost her. They were like lovers still, after all those years of marriage. They held hands and kissed, and my father was not above pinching her bottom when he thought no one was looking.

"Of course I want you to come, Mother. But I just couldn't ask you to do it—it's too much for you."

"So don't ask me to do it. I'm volunteering. I'll be there tomorrow. Your sister-in-law is picking me up at the airport in San Francisco and taking me to the hospital. David and Dad have been making arrangements since David got home a little while ago. And don't worry, the kids are fine. I talked to them both."

"Mother, did you say Bobby Sue is picking you up?" Bobby Sue was David's younger sister; a pretty, flighty girl who had moved to San Francisco some months ago. I had always liked her the best of anyone in David's family; she was cheerful, warm, and giving. But Bobby Sue reminded me of some lovely butterfly, flitting happily about, a breath away from disaster at all times. Flaky and always in some sort of jam, she seemed unable to stay with anything long enough to support herself. David's parents sent her money frequently, though they didn't like to talk about it. Sending

Bobby Sue Halper to pick Helen Rosen up at the airport was like making a chicken responsible for a deer.

"Yes, she promised to be right there at the gate when I arrive." My mother's voice revealed that she, too, wasn't sure Bobby Sue was dependable, which made her decision to come to California even more remarkable.

"Mother, keep the number of the hospital in your purse so you can call me from the airport in case . . . you feel like it."

"Oh, good idea." I could envision her relieved smile. "I'll be there tomorrow around noon. What should I bring? What's the weather like?"

"It's chilly and raining right now. Listen, you don't need a whole lot of clothes, Mother. Everyone is really casual here." Even as I said it, I knew it was wasted breath. My mother would be the same fashion plate at luncheon in the dining room at Rolling Green Country Club or dinner in the kitchen at Children's Hospital.

"Right," she agreed. "I won't bring much . . . besides I need room in my luggage for a few little things I have for Jobi."

I could imagine what the "few little things" would consist of, but I just laughed. "Mother . . . I'm so glad you're coming." I couldn't stop my voice from choking a little.

"I'm glad too, honey," she said softly. I could tell she was crying and didn't want me to know. Then my sisters, Leenie and Bonnie, and my brother, Larry, took turns on the line. They each expressed love and made little jokes to try to cheer me up.

"Don't let your mother loose in those San Francisco stores," warned my father, taking the phone last. "I'm sending her with a little change to buy anything you three need, and I'm afraid she'll spend it in the Minneapolis airport before she even leaves." I could hear my mother sputtering indignantly in the background, my brother and sisters laughing at my father's teasing.

112

"Dad, I don't need any money. I . . ."

"I'm sending it to you for safekeeping. If I leave it here, Leenie and Bonnie will weedle it out of me." Now my sisters chorused a reproach, and my brother guffawed loudly.

The warmth that was my family reached out and linked me back to their world. I hung up the phone at last and turned to look down the hospital corridor, my face set. A baby cried somewhere, and the odor of disinfectant drifted in the air. I walked down the hall toward the area where Paula told me I'd find the smoking lounge. I looked neither to the right nor left, and I listened to my brother's laughter instead of to the child who was moaning pitifully.

29

THE SMOKING LOUNGE TURNED out to be a hallway with delusions of grandeur. A widening of the corridor between two wings had been appropriated by smokers. A small battered couch and a few rickety chairs qualified the spot to be called a lounge, and two chipped ashtrays on a very early American coffee table proclaimed it property of an amazing number of smoking parents.

Emily was perched on a chair as I approached, dragging heavily on a cigarette. When she saw me, she jumped up and led me to another chair. The couch held two women and a child . . . one of the hairless waifs who wandered the corridors. Emily quickly introduced me to Lois, a fortyish woman with a suntanned, athletic body and short brown hair. Lois smiled and leaned forward to shake hands with me, and I could see by her eyes that I was not the only one who cried after dinner at Children's Hospital.

Lois, in turn, introduced me to a quiet woman with dark hair and eyes. Natasha smiled shyly and greeted me with a thick Russian accent. Obviously feeling left out, the chubby girl on the couch spoke up.

"Hiyah. Far out." I looked at her, and the smile nearly died on my lips. Puffy and without hair, as were many of the children here, this girl was different from any of the others. She appeared to be about ten, but as she put her blue-veined hand to her mouth and giggled mindlessly, I knew her chronological age didn't matter. The girl was retarded; that was apparent. But there was more to it than that. Her eyes didn't seem to focus and occasionally moved independently of each other. On the side of her head were strange markings in what appeared to be Magic Marker.

"Sarah, say howdy to Mrs. Halper," coaxed Emily.

"Far out!" repeated Sarah with great enthusiasm; then she rose and walked stiffly away. For the first time I noticed one of her legs was in a brace.

"Poor Sarah," murmured Lois, rubbing her tembles tiredly. Natasha shook her head sadly, but said nothing.

Emily saw my inquiring glance and explained about Sarah. "Brain tumor," she said briefly. "Two operations haven't worked and now they're tryin' cobalt. Poor li'l thing —she hasn't got much mind left anyway. Her mamma can't bear to come anymore."

"About all she can say is 'far out'!" Lois added. "Nobody knows where she picked it up—but she uses it to express almost everything."

I didn't know what to say. My throat felt tight again. I summoned a picture of my mother's kitchen table on Friday night. She was standing in front of it, my bauby beside her. They covered their eyes and intoned the rhythmic Hebrew words together. The candles they had just lit flickered in the old silver candelabra.

A teenage boy in a wheelchair joined the group in the smoking lounge. With one hand he pushed the large chair

114

wheels, the other firmly guiding an intravenous unit hanging from a stand on rollers. The bottle wobbled wildly as he pushed the chair, but the liquid maintained a slow steady drip into the thin tubing that led to his arm. I dropped my gaze and saw his right leg was missing from the knee down. Another of Dr. Wilbur's special problem children.

We had been told there were five children on the protocol study of osteogenic sarcoma at present. Four of them were boys, all older than Jobi.

This husky youth in the wheelchair was Carl. His brown hair was raggedly cut, his blue jeans and shirt faded and patched. But he grinned jovially and saluted with the hand taped to a board.

"Is your mamma comin' up this week, Carl?" drawled Emily.

"Naw," answered the boy cheerfully. "Three of the kids got the measles. So she ain't comin' here and the doc says I can't go home neither."

"Well, I should hope not. Measles will probably spread right through all eight kids, it's so contagious," interjected Lois. "And you know what could happen if you caught the measles, Carl."

"Yup," Carl replied with little concern. "It would kill me."

"It'll be me who kills you if you don't get your butt to the game room," called a tall, handsome teenage boy who had swung powerfully into view on crutches. His by-now-familiar-looking empty right pant leg proclaimed him as another osteo patient.

"Where are your manners, Michael?" asked Lois sharply. "Can't you say hello to everyone?"

Michael smiled sheepishly, his square-jawed, rugged face suffused with color.

"My son, Michael," introduced Lois, the reprimand in her voice now replaced with warm pride. Michael nodded pleasantly, but I noticed his left hand creep with supposed camaraderie around Carl's shoulder. He let his fingers slide down his friend's arm as the women continued to chat. Suddenly he grabbed a wad of Carl's abundant flesh and twisted it.

"Yeowch!" bellowed Carl. "What the . . ."

Michael's expression didn't change, and no one else seemed to have noticed the pinch. He smiled pleasantly and said, "See you folks later. Carl and I have a date in the game room."

Carl glowered and rubbed his sore arm. "Yeah, well I don't feel like goin'. Ya always beat me anyway."

Michael didn't reply. He appeared to maneuver his crutches to leave, but I saw he had also adjusted his fingers so his grip included some tubing from Carl's intravenous unit. Carl noticed immediately and wasted no time setting his wheelchair in motion to follow his friend down the corridor.

"Holy shit, Mike—I was comin'. Leggo of that!" Carl could be heard saying as the unusual pair of buddies disappeared around a corner.

"Those boys," chuckled Lois. "They're the terror of the ward."

"Yeah . . . exceptin' for when my Robbie's with 'em," Emily snorted. "Then they're worse."

"Like when they poured apple juice in all the specimen bottles that were sitting on the desk waiting to be taken to the lab."

We all laughed except Natasha, who barely managed a nervous smile. The poor woman looked as though she were about to jump out of her skin.

"I must go find Ivan," she said distractedly and quickly stood. Her skirt caught the edge of a box holding a jigsaw puzzle and the box tipped. Puzzle pieces scattered, and Natasha gave a moan of dismay. "I am sorry. Oh, I am so clumsy."

"It's nothing," said Lois gently as Emily and I quickly began to pick up the puzzle pieces. But Natasha's eyes filled with tears, and she fled down the corridor.

116

"Why did she get so upset over a puzzle?" I asked.

Emily sighed deeply. "It wasn't the puzzle, honey. Natasha is having a tough old time of it."

"She's a Russian refugee," Lois explained. "She and her husband waited a long time to come to this country. Then right after they got here, the bastard dumped her and took off."

"And as if it wasn't 'nuf to be alone in a foreign country, they just found out her son, Ivan, has Hodgkin's disease," Emily added angrily.

"How terrible for her," I exclaimed. "And to have to face it all alone . . ."

"She hasn't got any monopoly on that," said Lois bitterly. She looked as though she might say more, but Emily quickly changed the subject.

"Sharon's li'l girl is here for the same program as Michael."

"So I heard," replied Lois, squinting around the smoke as she lit a fresh cigarette. "That makes five with Carl and the other two boys."

"How long have the others been on the protocol study?" I asked.

"Carl's been on it for several months. He was diagnosed and operated on over at Stanford and they sent him right to Dr. Wilbur. Carl's doing really well." Lois paused and her eyes darkened. She exhaled smoke and put out her half-finished cigarette. No one spoke. Then she looked at me, tightening her angular jaw. Her resemblance to her son became obvious. "Michael wasn't quite so lucky. He was operated on in Oklahoma, back home. Then they sent us up to your country."

"Mayo Clinic in Rochester?"

"That's the place. They said there was nothing to do but radiate him with cobalt. So that's what they did."

There was a hollow feeling in my stomach. David had

117

told me all about Mayo's passive treatment of osteogenic sarcoma.

"So," said Lois loudly, trying too hard to be matter-of-fact, "the tumor spread to his lung, just as they promised. And now we're here."

"And Dr. Wilbur? What does he have to say?" I asked around my lumpy throat. Thank you, God, for sending us to Dr. Wilbur. What God? Thank you, David.

Lois smiled and blinked away tears defiantly. "Michael's the only one on the program who's disease has already spread, but Dr. Wilbur says we're going to try and lick it anyhow."

"I have tremendous confidence in him," I stated firmly.

"So do I, honey." Lois stared passed me out the dark window. "He's all we've got."

30

"DO YOU KNOW what's going on in that room across from the bathroom?" My mother's whispered voice was near hysteria. Her face was pale in the dim light filtering in from the corridor.

I stayed beneath the blanket and stared up at the ceiling. "Yes. I know."

"That little boy," she choked, "the fat one on the diet—they're all around him in that little room."

I didn't answer. What was there to say?

"Sharon!" my mother hissed. "They were pounding on his chest with their fists. Did you hear me? Pounding on that little boy's chest." Sobs were escaping her now. Jobi stirred,

118

but didn't waken. I sat up and pulled the distraught woman so she sat on the edge of my cot.

"Mother, don't cry in front of Jobi," I said, ignoring the tears racing down my own cheeks. "The boy is dying. I heard the commotion earlier. He has pneumonia. His lungs are so full of fluid, he's drowning."

My mother was breathing raggedly and staring at me in horror. I tried to soften my voice, soften the blow; but it only came out dull and flat.

"I told you when you got here this morning, don't look to the right or left when you walk down a corridor. Didn't I tell you that?"

She nodded woodenly. I hoped she wouldn't ask me how you could keep from listening to the sounds around you even if you didn't look. For that, I had no answer. Hours before I had lain awake in the dark listening to the little Mexican-American boy cry, his moans growing weaker as the night progressed.

"Please, nurse, please," he had begged. "Make me feel better." But no one could make him feel better. Not his grandmother, who sat in a chair outside his room, hands clasped and praying in Spanish. Pneumonia would do what leukemia hadn't managed yet. The leukemia cells were being knocked out by drugs, but so were the child's white blood cells—his body's only defense against disease.

It would be morning soon. Today Jobi would receive her first injection of Cytoxan, the first drug in the series. The protocol called for this drug to be taken every day for seven days. On the first and seventh days, a chemical called vincristine had to be injected with it. On the other days, Jobi could receive her Cytoxan in pill form—five pills at a time, to be exact. If she could swallow pills. Which she couldn't.

But I didn't want to think about that just yet. Not while the fat little Mexican-American boy who was on a diet lay dying.

My mother was quiet. She looked at me and at Jobi's sleeping little body, then out into the corridor where crepe-sole-footed figures kept running back and forth.

"There's nowhere here a person can cry," Helen said. Then she went back to her cot on the other side of Jobi's bed.

It was my mother's first night at the hospital. She had arrived that morning. My sister-in-law, Bobby Sue, was not at the gate to meet her, to no one's surprise. My mother had not panicked. She followed the signs to the luggage area and, in her cute blond way, found a nonexistent skycap to collect her mountain of bags and leave them on a cart by the exit. Just as my mother was about to consider panicking, she spotted Bobby Sue wandering around. Bobby Sue's giant sunglasses were perched atop moon-colored hair, and her long false eyelashes fluttered wildly as she looked frantically about for her lost in-law.

My mother called out, and Bobby Sue pounced on her warmly and triumphantly. A misunderstood airline name, illegible flight number, and sudden loss of memory regarding the time of arrival had not prevented her from picking up my mother at the airport as instructed.

My mother's arrival at the hospital was not without a certain dramatic flair. After profuse hugs and kisses were distributed to Jobi and me, she began to unpack a few things.

There were toys, games, books, and a new wardrobe of nightgowns and pajamas for Jobi.

"Grandma—kids don't wear pajamas and junk here." Jobi was not ungrateful, only honest.

"No pajamas in a hospital?"

"They like the kids to be dressed during the day," I explained. "That way it's not as though they're sick."

"And Grandma, ya gotta go to school here even if you're throwing up." There were times I wished my daughter weren't so graphic.

"They send sick children to school?" I still couldn't tell

from my mother's tone if she approved of all this information. She looked as though she might pick Jobi up and flee from the building.

"They have a school here at the hospital, Mom, and a teacher comes every day so the kids won't fall behind on their schoolwork."

"Isn't that amazing," she said politely, opening another suitcase. "Now show me where the refrigerator is." The suitcase contained provisions for a year in an air-raid shelter.

There were jars of chicken soup and bean with barley soup, two of my mother's specialties. Bauby had sent what appeared to be five pounds of chopped liver and a casserole of sweet and sour meatballs. Aunt Charlene's famous chocolate chip cookies, made especially for Jobi without nuts, joined the growing pile of food along with a Dayton box loaded with banana cake and brownies from Auntie Marcia. Uncle Frank's wife, my dear friend, Doll, had baked one of her wonderful homemade breads, in case the honey cake and kamish bread someone else in the family sent wasn't enough to round out mealtime.

I stared in wonder at the marvels emerging from my mother's suitcase. Jobi grabbed the cookies and ignored the rest. But it didn't really matter that she'd likely not eat the food. The little piece of herself that each woman had placed in the suitcase was for me more than the food was for Jobi. I understood that fact, and by the softening expression on my mother's face as she watched me touch the case lightly, I could tell she was satisfied I had gotten the message.

"When I left, Leenie and Bonnie were taking the children to a movie and Rita was at your house washing all their clothes from the trip," my mother added to the contents of the suitcase. "Now, Sunshine, you take me to this big kitchen I've heard so much about. I want to put all this away."

"Okay, Grandma. You have to label all the stuff with my name," Jobi said importantly. "I'll show you where everything goes."

"Later we'll go to that grocery store I saw across the street and get the other things we need," she told Jobi as they left.

I smiled and looked around the tiny room. The hospital bed and folded cots were submerged under a sea of luggage, bags, boxes, scattered clothing, and wrapped presents. My mother was here.

At dinner that first night, my mother had smiled politely at her plate laden with food of dubious origin. She frowned when she saw the way Jobi only picked at the food, and I saw her making a mental grocery list.

As we ate, she had nodded pleasantly at our chubby Mexican-American friend and his grandmother and scarcely blanched when Sarah came clumping through the kitchen on her brace, bidding everyone, "Far out!"

My mother didn't smoke, but she was happy to accompany me to the social mecca of the community, the smoking lounge. She and Emily were immediate friends, and when Emily discovered my mother could play bridge, her joy was unbounded.

"Now all we need is a fourth and we're gonna have us a li'l ole tournament," Emily laughed.

That night my mother met Lois and her handsome son, Michael, and the shy Natasha, and even Irene lighted briefly among us, little Chris clutching the hem of her waitress uniform. After Will Painter shook her hand heartily, my mother told me how pleasant it was to meet so many new people; how it wasn't going to be nearly as bad as she had expected. Of course that was before she woke me up because someone was pounding a little boy's chest.

31

WILL PAINTER'S WIFE, Lee Painter, arrived the morning after the little boy's death. It was very quiet in our wing. No one spoke of the tragedy, which made the empty room across from the bathroom seem emptier.

Lee Painter walked into the hospital and cheerfully destroyed the silence. Lee was a sanguine woman of forty with a stocky body and rosy, round cheeks. I took one look at her and knew she made good apple pies. Her giant husband saw her and gave a whoop, whirling her around. Lee blushed furiously, while a bouncy little girl wearing Will's face laughed and hugged them both. Jo Anna, a curly lock of brown hair hanging over solemn eyes, stood and watched her mother and father and sister.

Lee Painter pushed her husband away with a laugh and saw her elder child.

"Ah," she breathed. "Jo Anna."

Jo Anna flew to her mother then, to be wrapped in those generous arms. Then Will and the younger child pressed close against them and the family held each other for a few moments.

The scene had taken place in front of our room, and my mother and Jobi and I smiled at each other as the Painters moved down the hall toward Jo Anna's room.

Paula, head nurse, had suggested Jobi eat lightly that morning. I didn't find this worth mentioning to Jobi since it was the only way she ever ate anyway.

If my child was nervous about the injection she would

123

receive later, she gave no sign as she entered the kitchen with her grandmother and me. But earlier she had created a scene when a young woman in a lab coat came to prick her finger for a blood sample.

"Wait—wait!" Jobi had shrieked. "I'm not ready. I'll tell you when."

The young woman had chuckled and smiled and quickly made the tiny stab.

"We do this every morning here, Jobi," she explained. She pressed Jobi's finger to slides and allowed the trickle of blood to flow into several small glass pipes.

"You're lucky," the technician continued. "In other hospitals where I've worked, they draw blood from the arm to do all these tests. But Dr. Wilbur thinks you kids have enough needles in your arms without another one for blood. So we do just the finger stick."

"Why don't they do a finger stick everywhere if it's possible?" I asked, remembering the many times blood had been drawn from Jobi's arm in the hospital at home.

"Oh—it makes more work for the lab person. And probably they don't have a Coulter Counter. That little machine can do all kinds of tests from a very small blood sample."

Finished, the woman gathered her implements and left. As she moved down the hall, I heard Robbie Denton, freed now from lying on the gurney, run ahead of her calling, "Head for the hills! The vampire is comin'."

My mother, Jobi, and I decided to ignore the vapid-looking breakfast waiting in the kitchen. Grandma produced honeycake, and I salvaged the orange juice from our trays. The coffee was ready, as always, and Jobi happily sipped some coffee-flavored milk I fixed for her.

"Jo Anna and me are going to have a coloring contest today in O.T.," announced Jobi.

"That sounds good," I replied. "What's O.T.?"

"I don't know. Something payshunal therany. Jo Anna

showed me. It's a room and they have stuff you can make. It's really cool."

"Have another piece of honeycake, Sunshine," my mother coaxed. "Bauby made it especially for you."

"Uh-uh, Grandma. I'm full. I gotta find Jo Anna."

But before Jobi could gather her crutches to leave, we heard a child crying piteously. Will Painter passed the door, his face grim. He carried Jo Anna in his arms like a baby, her head on his shoulder as she sobbed. Lee and Jo Anna's sister followed them. They were heading for the treatment room. It was time for Jo Anna's chemotherapy to begin.

Emily had explained to me that one of the major problems facing long-term cancer patients was finding usable veins into which the drugs could be injected. After countless I.V. needles, the tired veins collapsed and could no longer support a needle. To a child like Jo Anna who had been on chemotherapy for a long time, a new I.V. needle meant the probability of a long torturous ordeal as the doctor attempted to find a usable vein.

When the Painters passed, I turned quickly to Jobi. "Hey —let's go show Grandma that store across the street. We'll just go for a little while."

Jobi looked at me. I could read no expression in her eyes. "All right," she said quietly. I would have preferred that she throw a tantrum rather than this silent acceptance.

"Did someone say shopping center?" My mother's face brightened.

I hummed the tune played at the opening of horse races, and Jobi gave a small laugh. My mother was famous for loving to shop. Years later, when a new shopping center called Ridgedale opened not far from her home, the family suggested it be renamed "Helendale."

"Okay gang—while we're over there we'll get coffee for our contribution."

"Yes," my mother agreed. "And one or two other things we might need."

125

We returned two hours later laden with my mother's "one or two other things." The shopping center was actually a rather long walk, and I was glad I had insisted Jobi go in a wheelchair. My own legs trembled with exhaustion, and I knew it would have been too much for a child on crutches.

My mother went to the kitchen to put our supplies away, and Jobi and I lay down together on her bed to rest. She snuggled into my arms, and I kissed her temple.

"Mom, when I get my I-Vee, will it hurt real bad?"

"I don't think so, honey. Just a stick, and then you won't feel the needle anymore."

"You'll be there, won't you?"

"You bet. I'm your Siamese twin."

"Maybe Grandma can come."

"If you want her."

"And Mrs. Beasly."

"Naturally."

Mrs. Beasly, looking a little worse for wear, was lying at the foot of the bed. She almost hadn't made it.

All packed and ready to leave on our trip to Disneyland and Hawaii, David, Heidi, Jonathan, and I had been in the family room waiting for our cab. Suddenly Jobi cried out from the top of the stairs.

"Mom! Mom! I can't find Mrs. Beasly."

I went to the bottom of the stairs. "Now, Jobi, she must be here somewhere."

"No. She's not." Jobi was crying harder now. "I've looked everywhere."

I went up to Jobi's room where Mary, our mother's aide, was searching for the missing doll.

"I really can't find it, Mrs. Halper," said Mary in distress.

"Everybody start looking," I called down. "Mrs. Beasly has disappeared."

"Dammit," I heard David mutter, as the other children raced about looking under cushions.

126

We looked every place we could think of, but the elusive rag doll remained lost. Jobi was crying and hiccuping, and David's face was getting very red.

"The cab's here," called Heidi.

"I can't go without Mrs. Beasly," wailed Jobi. "I promised her she could see Disneyland."

I drew David into the hall. "My God—I can't make her go to the hospital without Mrs. Beasly."

"Fine," spat David. "We'll cancel the trip and the drug program, and we'll all stay home and look for a doll."

I was ready to cry myself. Surely David understood how important the little doll was to Jobi. But his face hardened and he turned his back to me. He strode to the front door and ignored my imploring look.

"All right—everyone get into the cab. We're leaving right now or we'll miss the plane."

Quietly, the children picked up their carry-on bags and filed out of the house. Jobi, tears streaming, went past her stiff father on her crutches. They didn't look at each other. I called good-bye to Mary and followed the children. My father had gone ahead in his own car with most of our luggage and Jobi's wheelchair.

The drive to the Minneapolis/St. Paul airport took only a half hour. It was a very quiet half hour for a family on their way to Disneyland. Everyone stared out the windows at the patchy snow and pretended it was interesting. Halfway, the freeway took us near the exit to a major shopping center, Southdale. Suddenly, I had an idea.

"Driver, take the next exit and go past Southdale," I leaned forward to say.

"What for? What's the matter with you?" David turned from the front seat to look at me angrily.

"I have to get something," I said, waiting for him to explode. David was in no mood for side trips.

"You must be crazy!" he erupted on schedule. "We're on our way to catch a plane and you want to go shopping."

127

I usually backed off easily when faced with David's wrath, but everyone reaches the moment when a stand must be taken. "I wouldn't ask unless it was important. I have to run into Dayton's for just a minute," I insisted.

"Now I've heard everything," thundered my irate husband. The children cowered, afraid even to look at each other. The cab driver directed a questioning glance at David. He knew who'd be doing the tipping. David threw up his hand in the eternal gesture of male frustration and surrendered. With a sympathetic look, the driver entered Southdale's huge parking lot and pulled up to the curb in front of the department store I had named.

I got out of the car before David could hurl any more dark looks at me, and hurried into the store. It had just opened for the day, and there were few customers. I headed quickly for the toy department to a display which had caught my eye a few weeks before. She was still there.

A giant Mrs. Beasly doll, complete with blond hair and wire-rimmed glasses waited for me on a shelf. I grabbed her and fished my charge card from my purse.

"Charge it, and please hurry. This is an emergency."

"An emergency doll?" The saleswoman eyed me warily, but wrote up the sale.

I grabbed the paper bag from the poor woman's hand and shoved the doll into it as I hurried back to the exit. David didn't even look at me as I got into the backseat with the children.

"What's in the bag, Mom?" Heidi was the only one brave enough to ask.

As the cab headed for the airport again, I pulled the doll from the bag and handed her to Jobi. "Mrs. Beasly sent her great-aunt, Mrs. Sneasely, to keep you company until she comes back."

Heidi snorted and looked pointedly out the window. Jonathan was obviously disappointed my mysterious side trip

128

could be for anything as dull as a doll. Jobi didn't say anything.

"See, Sunshine," I prompted. "She looks exactly like Mrs. Beasly, only she's bigger. That way you can hug her harder."

Jobi gave me a sad little smile. "Thanks, Mom. She's nice."

My idea was a failure. Substitutes were not being accepted. I sighed and put my arm around my daughter.

We stayed in Disneyland for three days. Jobi set the new doll on top of a dresser in the hotel when we arrived, and there it remained throughout our stay.

On the third day, as we were repacking to leave for Hawaii, a bellboy came to our room.

"Package for Miss Jonie Halper," I heard him say to David. Everyone gathered around Jobi to see what was in the package. She opened it excitedly, and there, looking only slightly crushed from the trip, was Mrs. Beasly.

"She's here! Mrs. Beasly came!" shrieked Jobi, hugging the doll. Even Heidi seemed pleased, but perhaps she was only relieved it wasn't still another new present for her sister. David patted Jobi on the shoulder.

"But how . . . ?" I couldn't understand how the doll had arrived.

David looked a little sheepish. "I called home as soon as we got here."

"You called Mary? But why?"

"I thought the damn doll might have turned up by then. Sure enough, it had fallen between Jobi's bed and the wall, and Mary found it when she made the bed after we left. So I told her to send it here special delivery."

"David, that was one of the kindest things you've ever done." I laid my hand on his arm and would have hugged him. But that was enough sentiment for him to handle in one day, and he pulled away from me.

"Come on, you guys. Finish packing. We have to get going."

For once I didn't feel the flash of pain at his rejection of my affectionate gesture. I understood his need to keep his wall sturdy against the flood of emotion threatening him.

32

NOT LONG AFTER we returned from the shopping center, Paula came to get us.

"It's time to go to the treatment room," she said lightly. Jobi stiffened, and a look of fear crossed my mother's face.

I took Jobi's hand, but I kept my voice casual. I hoped my mother would take my cue. "Okay. This won't take long, will it? We were just going to start a new jigsaw puzzle."

"Oh, no," promised Paula. "It will only take a few minutes. You'll be at that puzzle before you know it."

"How can I work a puzzle with an I-Vee in my arm?" Jobi asked. Tears were only seconds away.

Paula knelt down so she could look Jobi right in the eye. "We're such experts here, after the I.V. is in, you'll be able to put a puzzle together faster than you can say Jack Robinson."

A dimple appeared in Jobi's cheek. "But it takes me hours to put one together now." Corn runs in our family.

"I told you we were experts." It must have run in Paula's family too.

Even my mother managed a bit of a smile as we headed for the treatment room. I tried not to look into the empty room across from the bathroom. The cries of the chubby boy still seemed to echo there.

130

Paula led us into the small treatment room and helped Jobi lie down on the narrow table. She pulled up a rolling tray of implements.

"I don't want to lie down," Jobi said suddenly.

"Well then, why don't you sit up," answered Paula. "Dr. Short will be here in a minute."

"Dr. Short?" I said with surprise. "I was expecting Dr. Wilbur."

"Dr. Short is Dr. Wilbur's assistant." She saw my distressed look, though I tried to hide it quickly so Jobi wouldn't become alarmed.

"Dr. Short is very good," Paula said emphatically. Then she leaned down toward Jobi's ear and said in a stage whisper, "But I can't figure out why they call him Dr. Short."

"What do ya' mean?" asked Jobi.

"You'll see," stated Paula mysteriously. Just then a white-coated young man entered. He was skinny and prematurely bald, had a prominent Adam's apple, and must have been well over six foot two inches tall. His loose-jointed movements reminded me of a crane I had once seen.

"Hello. I'm Dr. Short."

I suppressed my laugh and shook hands with him, as did my mother. Paula winked, and somehow Jobi succeeded in reducing her laughter to a small giggle. Dr. Short shook hands with her gravely and explained the procedure.

"Jo Beth, I'm going to insert a small butterfly needle into a vein in your arm. You'll feel a stick, and then you'll hardly notice it's there. Then I'm going to inject some medicine into the needle. But you won't feel that at all.

"Next, I'm going to let something like sugar water drip into the needle for a while. You need plenty of liquids, and that way we can make sure you get them even if you should feel too sick to drink anything later."

The careful explanation was given with little facial expression in nearly a monotone voice. Uh-oh, I thought. There must be one of these in every hospital.

"Do you have any questions?" Dr. Short asked politely.

Jobi shook her head and reached for my hand. I stood next to her.

"Now then, if you'll please lie down," requested the doctor coolly.

I was trying very hard to ignore my negative reactions to the man. It was hardly fair. I had just met him, and if he was Dr. Wilbur's assistant, he must be an exceptionally good doctor. But he seemed so full of importance and took himself so seriously. No smile had crossed his face since he entered the tiny room. Even his careful explanation to Jobi seemed by rote. I had the feeling he thought he had to work hard to be second to Jordan Wilbur.

Jobi clutched my hand. "I don't want to lie down. I want to sit up."

"All right," Dr. Short said smoothly. "But it's easier on you if you're lying down."

She looked at me and I nodded.

"Okay," she relented and lay back on the table.

Elastic was tied around her arm and pulled tight. The doctor regarded her veins for a moment and found one that pleased him in her hand. He wiped the spot with a swab.

"Dr. Short," I interrupted timidly. "If you put it in her hand, she won't be able to grip her crutches."

The doctor looked down at Jobi and surveyed her, as if noticing her missing leg for the first time. A flush of annoyance spread across his bald head, but he didn't look at me. He found another spot further up her arm.

Jobi squeezed my hand tightly, her eyes glued to the sight where the needle was to be inserted.

"Why don't you look at me, and it'll be over before you know it?" I suggested.

"No. I want to watch," she insisted. "I have to know how to do this when I'm a doctor."

I looked at my mother and raised an eyebrow in surprise. This was the first I had ever heard that my eight-year-old

132

daughter had chosen her future career. My mother shrugged back her mutual astonishment.

Paula was right about Dr. Short. He knew his business. The needle was in place with a good blood return before Jobi could complete the word "Yeowch."

"Are you done?" The future doctor asked hopefully.

"I just have to put the Cytoxan and vincristine in," Dr. Short replied. This was accomplished with little fanfare, and somehow my dread of the chemicals lessened when I saw how casually they were injected. I guess the playwright in me had expected a little more drama in the scene.

While the needle in her arm caused her no pain, Jobi was terribly aware of its presence.

"What if it falls out?" she asked, as Paula set up an I.V. drip.

"It won't," answered the nurse cheerfully.

"But what if it does?"

Paula sighed and smiled at the little girl. "If it actually comes out, which is unlikely, then we'd have to put it back in. But try not to worry about it, okay?"

"Okay."

My mother and I did our best to amuse Jobi the rest of the day. Jo Anna had had a very bad time with her treatment and did not come to play.

I ran into Emily once in the kitchen when I went to get Jobi some juice.

"How's it goin'?" she asked.

"So far she's doing great. Not sick or anything. Maybe she won't get any side effects."

"That'd be wonderful." The Southern lady smiled warmly. "Y'all never know."

"How's Robbie?"

Her smile disappeared. "His knees are still botherin' him. But say, listen. Maybe it's just growin' pains."

When Jobi went to bed that night, she said her tummy was hurting a little, but she fell asleep with no trouble. My mother and I were feeling almost smug about her lack of reaction to the drugs when we went to the smoking lounge to chat with Emily and Lois.

Lois told us her son, Michael, was finished with his first chemotherapy treatment, and they were going home soon.

"We'll be back in three weeks, though," she sighed. "I expect we'll see you and Jobi again then, Sharon."

"I'm not really sure. Jobi just started today, and I don't know when we can go home."

"I'm sure we can leave when Jobi's done with the medicines on the seventh day," said my mother confidently. She couldn't pronounce the names of the drugs, but she understood the general sequence.

"I'm hoping for that. I already miss David and the kids."

So much for wishful thinking. In the middle of the night, Jobi awoke and began to vomit violently. My mother jumped from her cot and ran to find a nurse. I held Jobi's damp hair away from her face and tried to support her trembling little body.

Two nurses I had never met ran into the room ahead of my mother.

"Cytoxan," pronounced one young woman, shining her flashlight at the mess in the bed.

"Cytoxan," agreed her companion grimly.

They deftly changed Jobi's nightgown without disturbing the I.V. unit and put clean linens on her bed. I pulled her hair high on top of her head with a band. Somehow I knew this was only the beginning.

My mother and I held a basin and sponged Jobi's face all night, as wave after wave of terrible nausea and stomach cramps attacked her.

She was given a suppository to control the reaction to the drugs, but it didn't help.

Throughout the agonizing night, when I wanted to scream and cry for her suffering, my child never once complained. She accepted this new ordeal as stoically as she had faced the other traumas life had hurled at her in the last three months.

After each bout of retching, she lay back against the pillows, her pale small face hardly darker than the linen. I smoothed the wisps of hair from her forehead, and she smiled a little, closing her eyes to sleep until the next bout.

33

WE HAD BARELY FALLEN asleep after Jobi's bout with Cytoxan when the hospital woke up. As in all hospitals, 7:00 A.M. at Stanford Hospital for Children meant shift changing, breakfast trays, and something new for us—doctors' rounds.

It seemed I had just collapsed wearily onto my cot and pulled the covers over me when the light in the room snapped on. I opened my eyes and started to sit up, muttering protest at the sudden brightness. But the sight that met my eyes caused me to pull the covers up to my chin, vainly seeking a place to hide in my skimpy cot.

Five men in white coats were crowded into our small room. They all peered with interest around Dr. Short as he read in a monotone from Jobi's chart.

"This is Jo Beth Halper, gentlemen. She suffered osteogenic sarcoma in November. . . ."

I peeked over at my mother who was clutching the covers around her with one hand while frantically pulling rollers and clips out of her hair with the other. I couldn't help laughing at the expression on her face—horror at being viewed in hair rollers by strange men and, always the lady, a polite smile.

Doctors' rounds were an almost daily morning ritual done sometimes as early as 6:00 A.M. Despite dozens of those eye-opening visits subsequently, I never got used to awakening to a group of fully dressed men staring down at me in my bed. Not that they paid attention to "roommates" of their patients. A tiny nod by one of the five or six doctors as they exited was the most acknowledgement given my nightgown-clad presence. Maybe that's what made me mad.

Dr. Short's troupe marched out of our room, and the "vampire" lady entered. I decided to give up on sleeping for that day. Jobi set up her usual shrieking protest to the finger stick. I wondered where she had found enough energy to make so much noise after her trying night. Personally, I was so tired they could have drained my blood with a fire hose and I couldn't have objected.

I left my patient mother to cajole Jobi into letting the lab lady prick her finger, and pulling on my robe, I headed for the bathroom. Fortunately, it was empty, because I got my period just as I entered the room and soundly and loudly cursed its one week early arrival. I had hoped to be home by the time it came, since menstruation meant inevitable cramps and depression for me. Depression—just what I needed in this place.

I went back to our room just in time to find my mother piling suitcases and bags onto a rolling cart.

"What's going on?" I asked her. "What are you doing?"

"We're moving," Jobi answered weakly but cheerfully.

"Moving? Where? Why?"

"I'm not sure," my mother answered wearily, taking clothes from the small closet where she had hung them only last night. "A nurse came in and said we were to move to another room."

Feeling angry and in a fighting mood, I stomped out of the room and went to the nursing station.

"Why do we have to change rooms?" I demanded of

136

Paula. "My mother just unpacked and we're tired out from a terrible night."

"Gee, I'm really sorry, Mrs. Halper. But you see we only use the little private room Jobi's in when a new patient first arrives or when . . . well, the point is, Jobi will enjoy a four-bed room. And so will you. There's lots more space."

"All right," I gave in. "Thanks, Paula." As I went back to help my mother repack, I wondered what Paula had started to tell me about the second reason for using a private room. Why did she hesitate?

A roommate might have been frightened by the invasion of Jobi, my mother, and me with all our possessions, but there was no roommate. The large, airy room appeared to be unoccupied. There were four hospital beds, two on each side of the room, with a folded cot next to each. Long windows made up one wall, allowing light to flood the room.

We bustled about putting our belongings away. That is, my mother bustled. Jobi dozed and I sort of slogged around. Coffee, I kept thinking wildly. If I don't get some coffee I'll do something evil.

A nurse entered carrying a glass of water and five pills in a paper cup. "Here you go, Jo Beth. This is your Cytoxan. Now don't forget to drink a lot today. Then you don't have to have an I.V. anymore."

Jobi looked at her doubtfully. She had never swallowed a pill before. I had tried to teach her many times using tiny children's aspirin, but I might as well have asked her to swallow Ping-Pong balls. The nurse didn't have any more success than I. After much gagging, choking, and five partially dissolved pills landing on the floor, we all gave up.

The pill problem was never resolved from that day forward. Every trick and innovation, some of them very creative, was tried by the nurses, but Jobi never learned to swallow Cytoxan pills. Instead, the pills were crushed and mixed with grape jelly, and Jobi had to eat the concoction with a teaspoon. It tasted awful, and it always took an hour of coaxing until she got it all down.

The next day we got our first roommate. Jobi had hoped it would be Jo Anna, but the Painters were all staying in the trailer and using the hospital as outpatients. Laurel Sardi, however, quickly made up for Jo Anna's absence.

All giant brown eyes and long shining dark hair, the six-year-old girl skipped into our room and plopped herself on Jobi's bed. She was followed by a thick-set man and a slight, pretty young woman with upswept hair, who scolded her for being a nuisance. Maureen and Nick Sardi had brought their daughter Laurel to Dr. Wilbur because X rays had revealed a growth on her collarbone. No one knew what was growing yet. Not so much as a biopsy had been done. But the Sardis' doctor at home in Salt Lake City had heard about Dr. Wilbur's success and sent Laurel to him without delay.

Maureen was a nervous young woman, though who could blame her? But she was cordial and friendly, and my mother and I both liked her at once. Nick had little to say, but seemed a pleasant man. Though they didn't speak to each other much, it was easy to tell Maureen was the dominant force of the pair.

Laurel ignored the adults, introduced herself to a weak but amused Jobi and convinced her to get out of bed and take her to the game room. Laurel's dark eyes took in Jobi's empty pants leg calmly as Jobi started out of the room on her crutches, and we could hear the two children blandly discussing Jobi's surgery.

Maureen, on the other hand, was deeply affected by the sight of my daughter. Her hand went up to her mouth in horror, and she sank onto Laurel's bed.

"What . . . what happened to her?" she asked.

I explained briefly, and Maureen nodded in misery.

"Osteogenic . . . however you say it . . . that's one of the things Dr. Wilbur said could be wrong with Laurel."

138

"He also said it could be only an infection or a dozen other things," Nick reminded her softly.

Maureen gave him a cold look and briskly began to unpack their clothes. She would stay here with Laurel, and Nick would remain in a nearby motel. Laurel was scheduled for surgery in two days. Whatever was growing on her collarbone would be removed.

Nick left, and my mother and I took Maureen to meet the smoking lounge crew. At almost any time of day someone could be found in the dingy hallway, either puffing away or working on a crossword puzzle, or both.

Emily and Lois were there. Lois looked jittery, a muscle twitching in her angular jaw, and Emily looked sympathetic.

"Is everything all right, Lois?" I asked hesitantly after introductions were made. I had noticed parents here rarely questioned each other on the condition of their children.

"Sure, sure," answered Lois brittlely, squashing out a cigarette and immediately lighting another. "We go home tomorrow."

"That's great," I said with jealousy. I was beginning to feel frantic to go home.

"Sure—great." Lois's eyes glittered. "Going home is great —if you have some big strong man to take you in his arms when you get there."

I wasn't sure how to respond to this. Both my mother and Maureen looked uncomfortable, as though caught listening in on someone else's conversation.

"I'm divorced, you know," Lois said flatly.

"No, I didn't know."

"Don't look so startled. Half the people here are divorced. If they aren't when they get here, they are before they leave."

"I don't understand," I said nervously. I didn't like this conversation. I felt badly for Lois, but I didn't want to hear about all of this.

139

"You mean the hospital has something to do with the divorces?" Maureen asked almost breathlessly.

"No, no o' course not," Emily broke in. "But Lois is right in a way. There's a lot of divorced folks here. No one's sure just why." She paused. Maureen looked pale.

Emily added gently, "Sometimes I think couples just can't stand the strain o' havin' a sick child."

"Yeah—my husband left somewhere between Michael's surgery and having his stitches out," Lois laughed harshly. Her bitterness was reaching out and trying to grab me.

It made me angry. I had David; we were closer now than ever. Lois and Emily were wrong. I thought about facing all this alone, without David. Or facing life without him. I shuddered and stood up.

"I think I'll go see what the kids are up to."

My mother and Maureen had had enough too, and they followed me back to our room. But I excused myself to them, too, and went to the phone.

"Mary? Hi—how's everything?"

Everything was fine, but then I knew that. I had spoken to Mary and the kids a few hours before.

"Is David home from work yet?"

He was there. Oh, thank you.

"Sharon? What's the matter? Is everything all right?"

"Yes—we're fine. Jobi's hardly sick at all anymore."

"Good—when you called again so soon. I thought . . ."

"I'm sorry. I just wanted to talk to you; just to say . . . hello. Y'know?"

"Are you sure you're okay?"

"I'm just having a bad period."

"Oh, that."

We laughed a little. David always described strange behavior on my part as my "menstrual personality."

"David, I miss you. I'm really homesick."

"Well, when do they say you can come home?"

"I don't know. As soon as Jobi's blood count returns to normal after the Cytoxan."

"So maybe by next week?"

"God—I hope so."

"Okay, call me in a couple of days and let me know."

"Right. David?"

"What?"

"Nothing. Kiss the kids for me."

34

WE STAYED IN THE HOSPITAL, my mother, Jobi, and I, for over six weeks. There were times I thought I would lose my mind.

I stood in the hall one day trying to pull myself together. Everything around me was wearing on my nerves, even my mother. I had snapped at her a few minutes before over nothing. So I piled guilt on top of my teetering load of emotions.

It was nearing the end of the second week after Jobi's first Cytoxan pill. In a little over a week it would be time for the next drug in the sequence. It was silly to be hoping we could fly home for just those few days. But I hoped and hoped.

A nurse pushed little Chris past me in a tiny wheelchair. His eyes were dull and lifeless. One scrawny wisp of hair still clung to his otherwise bald head. He didn't even bother to cry anymore when Irene left for her waitress job. Chris had given up.

I wanted to go home before I, too, gave up.

Restlessly, I wandered to the smoking lounge. Sarah was seated on the couch next to a fashionable young woman who was a stranger to me. Emily and Robbie were there too, Robbie in a wheelchair with ice packs on his knees.

"Sharon, honey, this here's Felice Brown," drawled Emily in her friendly fashion.

"Far out." Sarah beamed. She by now had lost all her hair from cobalt. The ink marks stood out vividly on the side of her head at the site of her tumor. She was getting fatter, I noticed, her face and belly blowing up from drugs. Her eyes were almost buried in her bulging cheeks, and her skin was a mottled bluish white. She was grotesque, and the sight of her made me want to weep.

Felice nodded politely to me and resumed staring out the window, blowing smoke in staccato puffs. Sarah began plucking at the sleeve of Felice's expensive-looking mauve suit jacket, giggling mindlessly. Felice jerked her arm away and moved farther from Sarah on the couch. I knew it must be embarrassing for a stranger to have to cope with Sarah for the first time, but I felt angry with Felice Brown for having been so obvious in her revulsion. Poor Sarah couldn't help what she was.

A hurt look crossed Sarah's face for a moment, her lip quivering slightly. Then her features returned to their slack, empty positions. With a chuckle, the child limped away, her brace squeaking.

"Is Sarah any better?" I asked Emily. Emily always seemed to know about the other patients.

"I'm afraid not," said Felice before Emily could answer. "My daughter will never get any better." She crossed her legs and blew smoke at the ceiling.

"You're Sarah's mother?" I asked in surprise. It didn't seem possible. This delicate woman looked like a fashion model, while Sarah . . .

"Yes," responded Felice. Then her voice softened. "Sarah

142

is my little girl." She stood, picked up her purse, and headed for the exit, her spike heels clicking on the floor. I never saw her visit Sarah at the hospital again.

Meeting Felice made me more depressed than ever. I felt as though I were living in a hole on the dark side of the world, a place most people didn't know existed. And I wanted to get out of it.

I longed for physical activity to help me shake off my dismal mood. I tried to go for a walk, but my period was still heavy, even after two weeks, and walking seemed to make it worse. Returning to our room, I passed the game room where Jobi was playing Monopoly with Laurel and some of the other children. I looked at Laurel's laughing face and felt a little better.

Laurel Sardi was one of the lucky ones. She didn't have cancer. How we all rejoiced when we learned that a benign tumor had been found on Laurel's collarbone. And how jealous some of us couldn't help feeling. The surgery had been performed at Stanford Hospital a few blocks away. Some of the bone had to be removed along with the tumor, but Laurel would be fine. Dr. Wilbur had assured Maureen her daughter's scar would be scarcely noticeable. Now Laurel was back at Children's Hospital to recuperate for a week or two, her arm in a brightly colored sling.

Jo Anna Painter and Laurel didn't seem to care for each other, so Jobi divided her time between the two girls. Playing with her friends and doing schoolwork took up most of Jobi's time, and she rarely complained about being in the hospital.

I didn't complain either—out loud. But inside I was screeching and howling. Jobi's white blood count had dropped, as predicted, following the Cytoxan. A normal count was around 5.0. Jobi's had dropped to less than .9. She wasn't allowed to leave the hospital grounds now, not even to cross the street. If she should contract a cold or flu, she would have no way to fight it. We couldn't go home until her body began manufacturing white cells again.

There came a bright sunny day, a rarity in Palo Alto in February. My mother got permission to take Jobi for a walk around the hospital grounds. Jo Anna was going too, and the girls carried on as though it were a major excursion. Jobi picked out her favorite outfit and asked me to brush her hair.

Tying her long dark blond hair in two ponytails with pink yarn ribbons, I leaned down and kissed the top of her head. I knew the hair might not be there much longer.

I had discussed the hair loss with Jobi quite frankly. While hair loss does not occur on every patient undergoing chemotherapy, it does on most. There was no point in offering false hopes to the little girl. Losing her hair would be bad enough without adding the elements of surprise and shock as well.

Dr. Wilbur insisted that all the children beginning chemotherapy must pick out wigs they liked and have them standing by. In this way, he felt they would get used to the idea of wigs before the need arrived and not have to suffer a moment of baldness unnecessarily. Of course, there were some children who didn't seem to care if they were seen bald. They owned wigs, but couldn't be bothered to put them on. I knew Jobi was far too vain for this to be true in her case. She would care very much indeed.

The wig man had appeared the day before. I was near tears at the sight of him and what he represented for my child, but I tried not to show my feelings to Jobi.

"What kind of hairdo would you like, Sunshine?" I asked as cheerfully as I could.

"My own," she said stubbornly.

I sighed. "I know, love, but you have to pick out a wig. You know that." I spoke gently and gave her a little hug.

"Mom, can't we find one that looks just like mine?" she begged desperately. I turned to the wig salesman.

144

"What do you have that's as clost to my daughter's hair as possible?"

"Ma'am, for children we recommend the short models. They're easier to manage and they come in smaller sizes. Now honey, how about this Shirley Temple wig? All the little girls like it."

He held up a brownish mop of short scraggly curls. Jobi made a face at it. He showed her a medium length red page-boy, and she turned her head away. Beginning to look annoyed at his resistant customer, the man pulled three wigs at one time from his bag. They were all variations of the short wig he had shown her first. Jobi's eyes filled with tears.

"I'm afraid none of those will work. Jobi wants long hair like her own, and that's what she's going to have," I stated firmly. "If you don't have the right thing, we'll have to look elsewhere."

With a resigned shrug, he took another wig from his large black case. It had glamorous long golden locks and was obviously meant for a grown woman. I was about to object when I looked at Jobi. The tears had been brushed away and an enchanted smile had taken their place.

"Oh, I like that one," she breathed.

I took the wig from the man's hands, ignoring his warning that it would be too big, and set it on Jobi's head. I tucked her own hair under the wig as best I could and handed her a mirror.

The wig was, of course, too big. The hair was also too long and full for Jobi's tiny face and much blonder than her own sun-streaked hair. But the part-line of the wig looked like real scalp, and that, combined with Jobi's pleased expression, settled the issue.

"We'll take it," I said.

"But, ma'am . . ."

"She likes it."

We concluded our business and the wig man left, muttering to himself. I wasn't worried about how Jobi looked in

145

the wig. I planned on getting one or two others for her later if she lost her hair. For now it only mattered that she like the wig and was accepting the fact she might have to wear it soon.

I had expected the wig episode to be more traumatic for both Jobi and me. That it wasn't, was likely due to the fact that the new wig lay in a box in the corner, and Jobi's own beautiful hair was still on her head, where it belonged.

35

"SARAH—WHAT'S THE MATTER?" I asked sleepily. The ten-year-old girl had been moved into our room after dinner the night before. Paula had confided in me that it was hoped that if Sarah spent more time with Laurel and Jobi, her mind, damaged as it was from the tumor, might be stimulated to function better. My mother and I had viewed our new roommate with some dismay. Sarah's grotesque appearance was disconcerting enough, but worse was the child's habit of wandering around the hospital and doing strange things— such as removing her clothing. The fact that Sarah's mother was continually absent meant she had to be watched by everyone else, and neither my mother nor I felt up to caring for another child. But we were ashamed of our uncharitable feelings and had decided to help Sarah as much as we could.

"Why aren't you in bed? It's only five-thirty." I tried to speak politely to the bloated white face being thrust in front of me.

"Far out," Sarah breathed a little morning breath at me.

A baby whimpered. "A baby?" I thought. "What next?" Then I remembered our other new roommates.

146

Late the previous night, a new patient had arrived. Maureen Sardi, my mother, and I had already gone to bed, and the children had been asleep for hours.

The sound of people trying to be quiet woke me. The wall-mounted light across from my bed had been turned on, and figures moved back and forth. The empty hospital bed had been replaced by a crib in which a small child now slept. Cots were being unfolded on either side of the crib by two women with the help of a night nurse. The older of the two had steel gray hair and wore glasses. I judged her to be about sixty. The younger woman was in her late twenties and had shining skin and wide-set eyes. Both women were attractive in a typically American middle-class way, and I wondered if they were mother and daughter.

I sat up in bed. The older of the women noticed I was awake and smiled.

"Hello," she whispered. "I'm sorry we woke you."

"That's okay. Don't worry about it." I got out of bed and approached them. The younger woman smoothed a blanket over her cot and turned to me.

"We hoped to arrive earlier, but our plane was late and we had trouble finding a cab." She sat down on her cot, obviously suddenly weary.

"I'm Sharon Halper."

"Kathy Peterson," the young woman greeted me. "And this is my mother-in-law, Winifred Peterson."

The older Mrs. Peterson touched my arm briefly. "Nice to meet you."

"And this is Amy." Kathy Peterson had indicated the sleeping toddler. The little girl turned her face and I could see rosy cheeks and fine curls so blond they were nearly white. I knew the closed eyes behind the pale lashes would be Scandinavian blue.

"We'll talk more in the morning," I had offered. I was tempted to ask about Amy. She looked the picture of health. But the middle of the night was no time for an exchange of tragedies. I was too tired and so, I was sure, were the women I had just met.

Kathy and Winifred were still asleep as I rolled away from Sarah's leer early the next morning. But Amy Peterson was beginning to stir, and I had a feeling the whole room would be awake shortly.

As I wearily put on my robe for the trek to the bathroom, my premonition proved correct. Eighteen-month-old Amy opened her eyes, took in the strange surroundings, and began to howl with fear.

Her mother jumped out of bed instantly and took the child from her crib. But even though Amy's sobs subsided into muffled sounds against Kathy's shoulder, the other occupants of the room had already awakened.

Jobi sat up and regarded the baby and Kathy curiously. My mother's eyes opened, and she looked about cautiously before sitting up. I knew she expected to see the team of doctors peering at her.

Kitty-corner from us, Laurel sat up with a grunt of protest and rubbed sleep from her eyes with a chubby fist. Maureen rolled over on her stomach and pulled the covers over her head. Sarah sat companionably on the edge of my cot and smiled at everyone.

"Far out," she welcomed the newcomers with a wave of her hand.

Winifred Peterson rose from her cot stiffly and went to Kathy's side to make comforting little cluck-cluck sounds at Amy.

Nine people in one room. I groaned inwardly. I knew the hospital was crowded, but I had not anticipated living the life of a sardine. I mustered a cheerful, "Good morning," as I hurried to the bathroom. Six varied greetings and a "Far out" followed me down the hall.

I decided to thank Sarah later for waking me so early. For once there wasn't a line of people waiting to use a bathroom stall. There were six stalls, but in the morning everyone had the same thought at the same time.

I washed my face at one of the many sinks and grimaced in annoyance. I had forgotten to slip my toothbrush in the pocket of my robe. I stepped out into the hall in time to see Jobi hopping down the corridor toward me, smiling happily, hair streaming.

"Why don't you use your crutches?" I admonished her, trying to sound stern as she flung herself into my arms.

"I told her," my mother smiled indulgently. Holding the battered pink crutches, she was close behind Jobi. "But she wouldn't listen."

"I think it's time for a new paint job," I said, firmly handing the crutches to my daughter.

"Oh—can I help paint?" asked Laurel Sardi eagerly as she joined us in the hall.

"Sure," said Jobi generously. "We'll do it in O.T. We can make dots and stripes this time."

My mother and the girls went into the bathroom, and I returned to our room in search of my toothbrush and some other toilet articles. Getting dressed in the morning required many trips to and from the bathroom. Space was limited and there was an unspoken agreement that no one would leave piles of belongings around the area.

Kathy was changing Amy's diaper, and Winifred was making up their cots as I entered our room. Paula had arrived and was trying to convince Sarah to relinquish her nightgown and put on her clothes. Maureen Sardi remained buried under her covers.

"There'll be coffee in the kitchen when you're ready," I told the Petersons. "The kitchen's just across the hall."

"Yes—we were there last night." Kathy picked up Amy and stood her up in the crib. "What do you say, Amy? Ready for breakfast?"

"Bott-o," crowed Amy, holding up an empty plastic baby bottle.

The Petersons headed for the kitchen, and I gathered my things. By the time I returned from the bathroom, still in my robe, but at least washed and brushed, the lab technician had arrived for the morning finger stick. Apparently I had missed Sarah's and Laurel's turns, because they each were holding cotton to a fingertip.

Jobi followed me into the room and spied the lab girl laying out tubes and glass slides on her bed. Jobi turned to flee, but my mother's entrance into the room thwarted her escape.

"Come on, Jobi. It only takes a minute," urged the lab girl.

"No—later. Do it later." Jobi's voice rose in panic. It was still hard to understand why this child, who stoically had endured major surgery and all its accompanying pain, cringed before a finger stick.

We coaxed her into sitting on the edge of her bed, and the usual argument began.

"Don't do it 'til I'm ready," Jobi commanded.

"Okay. You say when," agreed the lab technician, tiny pointed instrument poised.

There was a long silence.

"Well?" asked the technician.

"I'm not ready yet," explained Jobi.

"Come on, Jobi—I've got a lot of kids to do."

"All right. I'm ready."

The lab girl attempted to prick Jobi's finger. "Jobi—you said you were ready. Why did you pull your hand away?"

"I wasn't ready after all."

"Look, I'll make you a deal," the young woman said slyly. "If you let me prick your finger, I'll let you put the blood on the glass and make the slides."

Jobi thought it over. She looked at me for an opinion.

"Sounds good to me, Sunshine." My mother also added a nod of encouragement.

Laurel approached. "It doesn't even hurt," she said smugly, from the safe side of a finger stick. "Much."

Jobi scrunched up her face and stuck her hand out to the lab technician. Her other hand reached for mine. The tiny prick was over before she realized it had happened. Jobi uttered a belated "ouch," and set about making slides in a businesslike manner. Laurel watched with envy.

We went to the kitchen and investigated the breakfast trays. Lunch and dinner were sent on large platters and served family style off a long wooden table. But breakfast was individualized for each child; parents were on their own. I ended up eating Jobi's breakfast most of the time since she preferred Froot Loops when she ate at all.

I was so sleepy that morning that I was interested in nothing but coffee. My mother set the breakfast tray in front of Jobi, ignoring the faces she made at it.

"Come on now, dear. Get something into your stomach before you have to take the pills," came the grandmotherly advice. Cytoxan mixed with grape jelly would be Jobi's dessert after breakfast every morning that week.

We sat at a table with the Petersons and Laurel. Other people drifted in and out collecting trays. Many of the children were too ill to eat in the kitchen. Emily came for Robbie's breakfast, but only waved, not stopping to chat.

While still not an expert, I explained what I knew about the layout of the hospital to the Petersons. Neither of them smoked and didn't seem to be very interested in the location of the lounge.

"We won't be here long," explained Kathy. "Amy has to have five treatments this trip, and then we can leave."

"Is she having chemotherapy?" I ventured, hesitant to ask too much.

151

"No; cobalt," answered Winifred, removing her glasses because Amy had splashed some oatmeal on them.

"Amy has a tumor behind her right eye," Kathy said matter-of-factly. They wanted to operate at home, but we heard about Dr. Wilbur." Kathy sipped her coffee and turned to wipe Amy's mouth with a napkin.

"Dr. Wilbur is hoping to reduce the tumor with a special kind of radiation treatment and save her eye," Winifred picked up the story. "In Kansas City, they said she'd have to lose it."

"Isn't it amazing how many negative doctors are out there?" I gestured to the world beyond the hospital kitchen windows. Briefly, I explained Jobi's situation and our experience with doctors at home.

"But I have to admit," I added, "in the beginning my husband had to convince me to allow Jobi to be treated. I went along with the doctors who advised me to bury my head in the sand."

"So did I," agreed my mother. "At first it seemed better to do nothing rather than subject a child to more risk."

"I know," sighed Kathy. "The worst part about Amy's treatments is that she has to be put to sleep before every one."

"I didn't know cobalt was painful," I said in surprise.

"It isn't," Kathy said grimly. "But the patient has to be absolutely still if the radiation isn't to damage the eye itself."

Amy's grandmother lifted her from her high chair. The child wiggled to be set down.

"There's no way to keep her still except to put her to sleep." Winifred smiled as we watched the baby toddle about the kitchen.

"It's very dangerous to sedate a baby so often," Kathy said quietly. "But there's no choice."

After breakfast, my mother helped me give Jobi a bath. There was only one tub in the women's bathroom, and since Jobi couldn't stand on one foot long enough to have her hair washed in the shower, we grabbed the busy tub whenever it

152

was available. By the time we finished washing Jobi, her hair, ourselves, and most of the floor, I gratefully accepted my mother's offer to coax Jobi into taking her pills while I showered and dressed.

I made my first trip between my room and the bathroom carrying soap, towels, shampoo, cream rinse, deodorant, and lotion. After utilizing all this paraphernalia, I returned it to my room, wearing my robe and with my wet hair hanging. On my return trip I carried my comb, rollers, clips, and hair dryer. My last pilgrimage was for clothes and makeup. I am a rather modest person, so I usually dressed in the curtained shower stall, staying where the floor was dry, on the outer edges of the area. When the shower stalls were occupied, I dressed in a toilet stall, trying not to fall over the bowl.

At least my timing was good. I returned to our room clean and dressed just as my mother was praising Jobi for swallowing the last spoonful of her Cytoxan–grape jelly concoction. Jo Anna and Laurel had been watching the procedure and cheering Jobi on. The three girls left for O.T., happily planning a new artistic design for Jobi's crutches.

My mother and I changed Jobi's sheets. We didn't have to do it ourselves. But when the nurses were busy, as they were today in the overflowing ward, parents usually pitched in to help. We folded our cots to get them out of the way, and I left my mother to her shower marathon while I went to enjoy my first cigarette of the day.

I reached the smoking lounge just as the phones, which hung on the wall near the couch, rang. It was a community phone, and while not very private, it was better than the line at the nursing station which was usually tied up with hospital business. The lounge phone was a coin machine, but incoming calls were, of course, without charge. Outsiders usually called patients and their families on this phone, and whoever answered would feel obligated to search the ward for the person being called.

The call I answered was for Lois, and I walked down the corridor to her and Michael's room. Lois, carrying cigarettes, appeared before I reached their door.

"Phone for you," I called. She nodded and lit a cigarette as she walked.

I sat on the couch in the lounge preparing to write a letter to my friend Rita, who was helping my mother-in-law run things at home.

"Dear Rita," I wrote. "It took me two hours and ten minutes to get dressed this morning. Wouldn't you think I'd be gorgeous after all that time? But my hair is still too fine and I still have freckles."

I looked up from my letter to see a well-groomed woman gingerly seat herself on one of the rickety chairs.

"Hi," I greeted the stranger.

"Hello." She smiled tentatively. She placed a pink cigarette in a holder and lit it with a gold lighter. The woman wore a pale gray knit dress and matching suede pumps. Her hair was in a stiff pageboy style, and large gold earrings gleamed in her ears. As she lifted the cigarette to her mouth with a well-manicured hand, a huge diamond flashed at me.

When the silence deepened, I said, "I'm Sharon Halper."

"Leatrice Wellington," she said coolly. A pretty teenage girl approached and put a hand on Leatrice's shoulder.

"Well, Sydney." Leatrice's eyes softened. "This is my daughter. Sydney, this is Mrs. Halter."

"Halper. But call me Sharon."

Sydney had thick brown hair that swung from two pigtails. Curly tendrils decorated her hairline. She wore large-framed glasses that scarcely hid her thickly lashed hazel eyes. She smiled at me, her teeth even and very white, and then turned back to her mother.

"Are you ready?"

"Yes, dear. I've already brought the car around." Leatrice rose and smoothed the unwrinkled skirt of her dress. I wondered if she were attending a luncheon, bedecked as she was.

"Have you been to the Bullock's across the road?" she inquired. "Sydney and I both need new lingerie, and I'm told it's the only decent place to shop around here."

"I'm sorry—I haven't shopped there. I've only been to the grocery store to get Froot Loops."

"I see," Leatrice said after a slight pause. "Well, I suppose we'll see you later." She walked regally toward the door near the lounge with her daughter, nearly colliding with Irene, who was obviously late for work. Irene wore her waitress uniform, but had not removed two rollers from her hair. With one hand she groped for the rollers, with the other she munched on a piece of bread smeared with peanut butter. Somewhere down the hall, I heard Chris howling for his mother.

Leatrice viewed the younger woman with distaste and glanced down at her own dress to see if any peanut butter had jumped the short distance between them. She arched an eyebrow, but nodded slightly at Irene before preceding her out the door, propelling Sydney ahead of her. Through the window in the lounge, I could see Leatrice open the door of a sleek beige Cadillac for Sydney. Irene turned and widened her eyes admiringly to me as she passed the car.

I laughed and went back to the couch and my letter.

"I've never been surrounded by such an incongruous group of people all in one place," I wrote. "Where else would a waitress from Glendora, a society matron from Dallas, and a housewife from Golden Valley live in the same building?"

Lois, who had been conducting a low-toned conversation all this time, slammed the receiver back on its hook and sat in the chair.

"Kids," she muttered.

"Trouble?" I questioned politely.

"My daughter," Lois sighed, crushing her cigarette vehemently in an ashtray. "I don't like to leave a seventeen-year-old girl alone, but what am I supposed to do?"

155

I shrugged helplessly.

"I think she's got a boy shacked up with her there. So I told her to get her butt down here right now. She can stay with Michael and me for a while."

"When is she coming?" I asked, not knowing what else to say.

"I told her to get on a bus tonight and then I hung up before she could argue."

"Lunch," someone called down the hall. "Come and get it."

"I'd better go find Jobi," I said, relieved for the excuse to leave. Lois seemed to consistently involve me in discussions that made me uncomfortable. "She'd never eat if I didn't insist," I added to my excuse for leaving.

Lois nodded. "I'll catch up with you later."

My mother was glaring at our room when I returned.

"What's the matter?" I asked her.

"I didn't realize we'd have to live out of our suitcases permanently. How are we supposed to keep the room neat?"

I surveyed our nine-bed dormitory. Open suitcases lined the floor. Folded cots leaned against the walls with pillows and extra blankets stacked on top of them. The children's bedstands were covered with bottles, jars, crayons, and toys, and the windowsills were piled with cards, plants, and packages of all kinds. My mother was right. The room was a mess.

"I have a great idea, Mother. Let's not look at it."

I coaxed her out of the room and out into the hall. The children were returning from O.T., and we all went into the kitchen for lunch.

Maureen Sardi had finally awakened, and she and Laurel sat at the table with us, as did the Painters. Nearby, Carl and Michael were haggling over a bag of potato chips. Robbie Denton entered the room with Emily and solved the problem for his friends by grabbing the potato chips and fleeing. Carl and Michael, one in a wheelchair and the latter on crutches, had little hope of retrieving the stolen goods.

156

Emily shook her head, but couldn't help laughing as she sat down next to me. "That boy o' mine has the devil in him. That's for sure."

"How's he feeling?" I wondered.

"When he doesn't complain, ah don't ask."

After lunch was schooltime for everyone who could get there. The small school building was across the grounds from the hospital, and the modes of travel to reach it were varied. For those who couldn't walk, there were wheelchairs, gurneys, and crutches . . . most of these spurned by the students, who preferred more interesting transportation. Most popular were scooters, tricycles, and wagons.

Today Jobi opted for a red wagon. She jumped in it and chose my mother to do the pulling. Jo Anna Painter, solemn as usual, held her hand and walked alongside. Jo Anna's father had told me that while she had always been introverted, there was no question that her illness was causing Jo Anna to withdraw further into herself. Will was pleased at his daughter's burgeoning friendship with Jobi. When Jo Anna spoke, it was usually to Jobi.

The weather was still being kind. The sun shone warmly and the sky was clear and soft. At home, during rare moments when the snow melts, grass and bushes are shriveled and brown at that time of year. In California, there was green to be seen, and it made me feel good, so I went along for the walk despite my continuing menstrual problems.

The path to the building that housed the school twisted and turned among trees and gardens. The hospital grounds were beautiful, and there was a playground with swings and a sandbox for the children.

My mother and I left Jobi with the young teacher. Jobi's teacher from home had packed a box filled with books and lessons and sent them to us, so there were strong guidelines for the hospital teacher to follow.

The older boys entered the building as we left, and I

157

wondered if the "unholy three" terrorized the schoolroom as much as they did the oncology ward.

I sat down on Jobi's bed to finish my letter to Rita. My mother was searching for a book among the bags and boxes, when Maureen came to tell her she had a phone call.

I learned later the call was from my father; one of many calls he made to express his loneliness for her. My mother didn't tell me about his almost daily call until years later. She didn't want me to feel guilty for keeping her away from home.

"I'm back from lunch and probably fatter," I penned to Rita. "The food here reminds me of the lunches served in the cafeteria at North High. Remember? Chow mein that was ninety percent cornstarch and ten percent vegetables. One slice of roast beef accompanied by spaghetti, corn on the cob *and* mashed potatoes.

"To tell you the truth, I think much more about my family than the food. Heidi and Jonathan are on my mind all the time. How I wish I could hug and kiss them just once. Do you think they're all right with me away all this time?"

I finally finished my letter, and my mother and I walked back to the school building to fetch Jobi. The children were exiting as we approached, and the beauty of the day seemed to have put them all in high spirits.

My mother found Jobi's wagon, but before she reached the door of the building, Jobi came hopping out, Jo Anna and Laurel behind her.

"Here's your limousine," my mother gestured to the wagon. "How was school?"

But Jobi neither answered nor climbed into the wagon. Laughing joyfully, she hopped across the walk and onto the grass. She and the other two girls sat down and began rolling about, giggling. Laurel's movements were only slightly hampered by the bright blue arm sling she wore.

I stood and watched them, smiling at their fun, but my

158

mother pulled the wagon onto the grass, following Jobi. Jobi stood as my mother approached her, but instead of sitting in the wagon, she began doing cartwheels away from her grandmother. I couldn't help but laugh at the sight of my mother chasing after Jobi, arms outstretched, obviously trying to catch her if she fell.

My mother took Jobi to the kitchen, hoping to persuade her to drink some fruit juice and begin diminishing the stockpile of food from home. I saw the Petersons had returned from Stanford Hospital. Amy was asleep in her crib, ink marks similar to Sarah's visible on her head. Winifred was unfolding her cot for a nap of her own. Kathy saw me and came to chat in the hall.

"How did it go?"

Kathy looked exhausted. She pushed her hair off her face wearily.

"Okay, I guess. She screamed her head off when they gave her the shot to put her to sleep, but I suppose that's not strange for a baby."

I laughed and reassured her. "Jobi's eight years old, and she carries on like a banshee when they do a blood test on her."

"They had a little trouble waking Amy up after the treatment," Kathy said, trying to be casual. "They're going to adjust the dose tomorrow."

"How about some coffee?" I suggested.

"Thanks, but I think I'll join the family nap." She indicated her mother-in-law and daughter. "Winifred has been great. But she's not so young, and this is a real strain on her."

"How nice that your mother-in-law feels so close to you . . . to share this with you, I mean."

"Yes. I know it's unusual, the relationship Winifred and I have. But she's such a reliable, you-can-lean-on-me person. My own mother's at home swooning over the whole thing."

"I never believed my mother was very strong either," I

159

said thoughtfully. "But she's really come through for me since Jobi's surgery. I don't think *she* knew she had it in her."

Dinner that night surpassed itself in blandness. As everyone sat at the tables picking at dry turkey slices under sticky gravy, Irene suddenly stood up and banged her spoon on her glass. Everyone stopped talking and looked at her in surprise.

"Hey," Irene, still in her waitress uniform, protested. "I can't eat this tonight. Who's for a super duper everything-on-it pizza from Tony's?"

There was a moment of silence and then an outburst of enthusiastic response.

"All right!" cried Carl, hoisting himself out of his wheelchair so he could stand and be heard.

"Make sure there's plenty o' sausage," demanded Robbie.

"Hold the anchovies," was Michael's request.

"Boy, does that sound good to me," commented Lois.

"Okay, how many want in?" Irene, with a professional air, whipped out the order pad from her uniform pocket.

Nearly everyone in the room ordered pizza. It became too complicated to figure out so many individual orders, and it was finally decided that four extra large pizzas with "everything on them" would be ordered.

"Uh-oh," remembered Irene. "No delivery from Tony's on week nights. "Who's got a car here?"

No one in the room did. Faces became long with disappointment. Then a cultured voice was heard from a corner.

"I'd be happy to place my car at your disposal."

At one of the few small tables sat Leatrice Wellington and her daughter, Sydney. I had learned from Emily that Sydney was one of Dr. Wilbur's Hodgkin's disease patients and was at present doing very well. She was in the hospital for a treatment that would begin the next day. Emily had told me Sydney was a pleasant, friendly girl, but her mother kept them both at arm's length from the other patients and their families.

Tonight Leatrice had changed her clothes for what she

160

must have thought was suitable dinner attire. Her knit dress had been replaced by black wool slacks and a white silk blouse. She might have been entertaining at a small intimate dinner for four instead of offering to drive to Tony's to get pizza for twenty.

The pizza was thick, gooey, spicy, and wonderful. Strings of hot cheese slid down over pale little childish faces and healthy but worried grown-up faces alike. Leatrice Wellington leaned over to wipe tomato sauce off Chris's face. Natasha, the Russian immigrant, tasted her first bite of American junk food.

"Not like Russia," she pronounced. We decided that meant she liked it.

The pizza spirit lasted beyond dinner, and the children responded enthusiastically to an invitation to play bingo in the game room. Some of the parents went to watch, but I headed for the smoking lounge.

Lois, Emily, Maureen, and I sat and talked about nothing; marking time until the children would go to bed and our nightly bridge game could begin. At such times, when we smoked and gossiped and played cards, it was possible to forget why we were there. As long as we were careful to say nothing to remind ourselves. And as long as no child cried out.

36

THE DAYS PASSED. I read, crocheted, and my mother, Emily, Maureen, and I played bridge unendingly. The four of us became as close in those weeks as friends of years' standing. We learned a great deal about each other, and did a lot of leaning.

I knew that Emily's husband, Dan, was in tobacco, and their marriage was like a rock. The Dentons had five children besides Robbie, all girls.

Maureen's husband, Nick, was a bank teller in Salt Lake City, and their marriage quivered like Jell-O.

"I don't like him to touch me," Maureen had confided in me one day. "I don't know why. We've been sweethearts since our high school days. But since Laurel was born, I just can't let him . . . you know."

No wonder poor Maureen had blanched when Lois talked about the divorce probabilities in the hospital. It had hit too close to her home. And mine?

One night, long after the children had gone to bed, Emily was late in joining us for cards. Lee Painter had come in from the trailer to kibitz, even though she didn't play bridge. Lee sat comfortably in an extra chair, knitting, while Maureen, my mother, and I waited at the card table. When Emily arrived, she seemed shaken.

"Is there anything we can do, Emily?" my mother asked warmly.

"No, no big thing. It's just that Robbie and Carl have been rooming together and Carl's goin' home tomorrow. There are a lot of patients leaving now, so they want to

162

close off the ward Robbie's in and have him move to one o' the private rooms."

Lee looked up from her afghan. "How did Robbie react to that?"

"Like he was bein' boiled in oil." Emily chuckled a little.

Lee smiled sadly. "Can't say I blame him."

Maureen looked at me questioningly. I shrugged, but then I remembered Paula stammering over the use of the private rooms.

"What's the story on these rooms?" I finally couldn't help asking. "Why does everyone speak so ominously about them?"

Lee looked down at her knitting, her plump fingers flying faster, though she closed her eyes.

Emily looked at me and tried to smile. "It's like Robbie says . . . , 'I ain't goin' to one of them little rooms. That's where they put you when you're dyin'.'"

Suddenly I understood. The Mexican-American boy had been put in the small room the night before he died.

Lee looked up. "The kids think once they go into one of those rooms, they never come out."

37

A FEW DAYS LATER, Jobi's blood count had not improved. We would obviously have to stay through the next treatment. Worried that the hospital was too much for my mother, I tried to convince her to go home without us. She refused. I knew she was beginning to worry almost as much about me as about Jobi.

I continued to bleed, the flow becoming heavier each day.

Listless and tired all the time, I finally asked Paula if she knew of a gynecologist in the area. I explained to her about having my period for weeks, and she arranged for me to see a Dr. Brighton the next day. The hospital solicitously sent me there in the van used to transport patients between Children's Hospital and Stanford Hospital, where tests and surgery were done.

Dr. Brighton was kind and reassuring and could find nothing to explain why my period wouldn't go away. He gave me birth control pills to take, explaining that the same hormone that prevented pregnancy might also stop the bleeding.

I took one at bedtime, laughing a little. I had had a tubal ligation after Jonathan was born because all birth control methods, including pills, had failed to work for me. Now here I was taking the same brand of pills I had used when I became pregnant with Jonny.

I became abruptly and violently ill. It was like a repeat performance of Jobi's Cytoxan act, only now I was the one writhing in my bed and moaning with cramps and nausea.

I decided I'd rather bleed forever then become so ill from birth control pills again. So I didn't take any more and the next day I bled harder than ever.

Then one afternoon my cousin Paul came to visit. He had borrowed a car from a friend and driven to Palo Alto from San Francisco. We were delighted to see him, ponytailed hair, unkempt beard, and all.

Paul's wife, Cindy, had sent a special soup she made for Jobi. Paul said it was made from vegetables and kelp and other nutritious things, and he actually convinced Jobi to eat a bowl of it. She made faces, but couldn't refuse her adored cousin.

When Jobi left the kitchen to find her friends so they could meet Paul, he turned and gave me a searching look.

"What's wrong with you?" he asked. I knew it was pointless to evade those deep eyes, so I told him about my bleeding.

He smiled and told me not to worry. "Wang can help," Paul reassured me.

"I'm afraid Wang can't do anything about this, Paul." I tried to hide a smile at the thought of a Chinese spirit discussing my menstrual period. "Besides, I don't want to leave Jobi to drive to San Francisco for a reading."

Paul smiled again. "Wang often does readings for people who are far away. I'm sure he can handle Palo Alto from San Francisco."

"All right. Why not." I was glad my mother wasn't in the room. I didn't think she would understand about Eldon Gunderson and Wang. I wasn't sure I understood myself.

I had barely gotten dressed, when Paul arrived at the hospital the next morning.

"Paul—what are you doing here?"

"Wang did your reading last night."

"You're kidding! That fast?" I didn't really believe in all this. It was more like a game.

Paul grinned. He knew exactly what was going through my mind.

"Come on, Sharon. Put on a coat or something; it's raining."

"Why? Where are we going?"

"I'll tell you on the way," Paul promised. "We'll be right back."

I told my mother I was going out with Paul for a little while. She looked puzzled, but didn't question me.

Paul and I got into the battered car he borrowed from his friend. Rain spattered on the windshield, and the inside of the car smelled damp and old.

"Hey—where are we going?" I demanded.

"To a shopping center."

"Wang told you to take me shopping?"

He laughed. "Wang said you have a severe vitamin deficiency. You've been under a lot of stress and your diet isn't giving you what you need."

"What? You mean the delectable cuisine in this hospital is inadequate? Impossible!"

This time he didn't laugh. "It's true. At stressful times your body needs more of certain vitamins and minerals to help you cope. Wang gave me a specific list."

"Paul, do you seriously believe just taking some vitamins will stop the bleeding?"

"Yes." If there was room for doubt in my faith in Wang, there was none in Paul's.

Paul selected the vitamins in the health food store from the list he said Wang had given him, including kelp tablets.

"Seaweed?" I giggled.

"Wait and see," he said firmly.

Paul dropped me back at the hospital. He was in a hurry because his friend needed the car.

"Take them in the doses I wrote down. I'll see you soon." He left before I could argue.

Telling myself it was all nonsense, I took the pills. My mother saw me swallowing some kelp tablets that night and questioned me.

"What are those strange green pills you're taking?"

"Kelp."

"I beg your pardon?"

I decided to tell her the whole story of Eldon Gunderson and Cara and the spirit, Wang. I thought she'd laugh at best, or more likely, think I had lost my mind. Ladies who golf at the country club and attend fund-raising luncheons for City of Hope don't believe in spirits.

But again, Helen Rosen surprised me. She looked thoughtful after I finished telling her about the first and second readings Wang had done for me.

"He called Jobi 'Sun'?" she asked, frowning.

"Yes. That got me, too."

166

"And these pills Paul gave you—can they hurt you in any way?"

"I don't think so. They're just vitamins."

"So take the pills. You never know." An echo of my own philosophy these days.

Three days later, my bleeding stopped. It didn't just slow down, it stopped completely.

"I can't believe it," I said joyfully to Paul on the phone.

"Believe it," he replied. I could almost see his warm smile, his eyes crinkling.

"Paul, I know Eldon doesn't ask for money for readings, but I feel as though we should . . ."

"David sent Eldon a donation a few days ago. Eldon and Cara used it to buy books to give to some of the people who come to them for help."

"David did that?" David sending money to Eldon Gunderson was more incredible than my period stopping.

"We'll make a believer of him yet," chuckled Paul.

I didn't know whether either David or I believed in spirits, but to this day, we both take vitamins during times of stress.

38

HOW WONDERFUL THAT my bleeding had stopped. How unfortunate that my depression remained. My need to go home became a tangible thing. I was obsessed with leaving the hospital. It was everything I could do to keep from taking Jobi and running out of the building.

The time came for Jobi to receive the second treatment on the protocol. For some reason, high-dose methotrexate was the drug I most dreaded. It would be administered in an

I.V. drip, then a so-called rescue, Leucovorin, an antidote-type drug, would be given every four hours over a twenty-four-hour period. The rescue was given to reverse the lethal effects of methotrexate. It was also necessary for the patient to drink great quantities of liquid during the twenty-four-hour rescue period.

But Dr. Wilbur assured me I didn't have to worry about lethal doses and rescues. His staff was well trained, and there would be no problems they could not handle. He gave me other things to worry about instead. Possible side effects from methotrexate included severe sores in and around the mouth, damage to the teeth, and possible eye problems. I was told to make sure Jobi was seen by a dentist and eye doctor regularly.

My mother, Mrs. Beasly, and I helped Dr. Short start Jobi's I.V., as we had the first time. Again, he had no trouble. With trepidation, I watched the yellowish liquid drip into her arm. The color of it looked evil to me.

Methotrexate made Jobi even sicker than Cytoxan. While the needle could have been detached from the bottle between rescues by using a heparin lock, she was too sick to walk around anyway. She remained in bed, the rescue being injected directly into the needle in her arm, saving her from additional sticks. Jobi claimed she could taste the rescue drug.

"It tastes like rotten fruit in my mouth," she protested.

"Could it be?" I asked the nurse who had injected it.

"Who knows?" she shrugged. "Around here anything is possible."

Later in the day my nerves and my habit could stand it no longer. Leaving my mother to sponge Jobi's face for her, I headed for the smoking lounge. As I passed along the corridor, I heard the wail of an infant. There were no small babies in the hospital that I knew of, but the sound was unmistakable. It came from the last room before the smoking lounge.

I looked in and saw Dr. Wilbur and a young couple standing around a crib. The couple appeared to be in their early twenties, the girl in faded jeans, her hair in long braids with beads and yarn woven into them. The young man also wore jeans, and he had an earring in one ear.

Dr. Wilbur noticed me and beckoned me into the room.

"Sharon Halper, I want you to meet Phyllis and Ray Arness. They just arrived."

I greeted them and walked over to the crib. The two young people barely smiled. I could tell they were terrified.

"And this is Quinta." Dr. Wilbur smiled, looking into the crib. In the crib was a newborn infant, spindly arms waving frantically. So tiny; so helpless. And dying of leukemia.

Later, after I had coaxed her out of the baby's room to get some coffee, Phyllis told me about Quinta. First I peeked in on Jobi, who was dozing along with her grandmother, then I joined Phyllis in the kitchen. She told me Ray had left to go back to his construction job.

"He was out of work for a long time before he got this job, so he doesn't want to lose it," Phyllis said nervously. "He got the job a couple of weeks before Quinta was born." Saying Quinta's name made Phyllis start to cry.

"We only got married because she was coming. We were living together a whole year before I got knocked up, and we were doing fine. But we thought, for the baby's sake . . ." The distraught woman blew her nose and slurped coffee from the cup I pushed toward her.

"Now they say my baby's got leukemia—acute, they called it. She could die." A fresh wave of crying overcame her, then Phyllis said, "But they say this Wilbur guy is good, huh?"

"The best," I answered and patted her arm.

Quinta's leukemia was so far progressed, they began her treatment that very day. The I.V. needle was placed in a vein in her head to keep it safe from her flailing little arms

169

and legs. Phyllis was frustrated because she couldn't hold her baby properly with the I.V. setup.

Ray returned to the hospital that evening accompanied by an older man. I didn't know who the man was, but when I passed Quinta's room later on my way to the smoking lounge, I heard strange mumblings and incantations. I couldn't help looking in. Ray stood near the bed, his arm around Phyllis. The older man was there wearing some sort of vestments, and there were candles lit. The man muttered and began invoking the Lord to come to Quinta's aid. He laid his hands on the tiny baby and she shuddered.

I quickly backed out of the room, feeling like an intruder. Phyllis found me in the lounge a few minutes later. She seemed more relaxed and smiled for the first time since I met her.

"That was the Reverend Peter Elmquist," she said, her eyes shining. "He's a faith healer, and he's going to keep coming until Quinta's well."

"That's wonderful, Phyllis." Who was I to scoff? "Does Dr. Wilbur know about Reverend Elmquist?"

"Oh yeah, for sure. He said he wouldn't object to anyone we want to bring in. Dr. Wilbur said he believes in trying anything that might work. He said stranger things than faith healers have been used around here."

Eldon Gunderson's face, slack, with eyes closed, flickered through my mind. I heard the voice of Wang say, "There is one in a high place who believes as we do."

Dr. Wilbur?

When Ray showed up with a machine to make carrot juice for Phyllis to feed to Quinta—at the advice of Reverend Elmquist—and Dr. Wilbur said it was fine with him, I decided, yes . . . Dr. Wilbur.

Jobi's nausea slowly disappeared; the rescue had done its work, and the I.V. was removed.

170

"Can we go home now, Mom?" Jobi asked anxiously. She was becoming as homesick as I, moping about.

"I hope so, love. I hope so."

But when the lab reports came up, the news was bad. Methotrexate did not affect the white count, but the Cytoxan hadn't relaxed its grip on Jobi. Her white cells still counted a low .9.

"Well what does it have to be before we can go home?" I practically shouted at Dr. Short.

"Now, now, Mrs. Halper." His Adam's apple bobbled in disapproval. The doctor admonished me in a patronizing tone. "Surely you care more for Jo Beth's health than your own desire to leave."

Why you sanctimonious bastard, I thought. Who are you to question me on how much I care about my daughter's health? But I didn't say it. My mother must have sensed how I felt, because she quickly came to my defense.

"Doctor, we're all anxious to go home. We've been gone a long time, and my daughter has two other small children. But naturally, we wouldn't do anything that could hurt Jobi."

"Well, your attitude about going home is not what it should be," Short sniffed.

Instead of strangling him, as I gleefully envisioned, I repeated tightly, "What does her white count have to be so we can take her home?"

"I'd say at least 2.0," he said, leaving the room.

"How long will it take to get there?" I followed him down the hall.

"I really can't say. Ten days . . . two weeks . . . maybe longer. I just can't say." He gave me a disapproving glance as he entered another room.

Two weeks. No, it wasn't to be tolerated. It had been a month since I had seen my husband, my children; six weeks since I'd been home.

I sank down onto the couch in the smoking lounge and

started to cry. I hoped no one would show up until I pulled myself together. Everyone here had something to cry about. So who was I to lose control? But I couldn't help it. I was overwhelmed with bitterness and self-pity.

A shadow fell between me and the long windows I faced. I looked up and there was Paul. He sat down next to me and handed me a handkerchief.

"Thanks," I snuffled. "I was just about to use my sleeve."

"What's bothering you?" he asked. "You're really up-tight."

"Does that mean I'm a nervous wreck?"

Paul nodded. "Something like that."

I told him that we still couldn't go home because of Jobi's blood count and that I was falling apart.

"Hey, listen," he said, touching my hand. "Cara wants to see you."

"Cara? Eldon's wife? Why?"

"She told me a while ago to bring you there. She's been worried about you." Paul touched my hand.

"Let her worry about Jobi. She's the one with the problem." I liked Cara, but I was in no mood to go visiting with so much on my mind.

"Sharon, you've got a problem, too. Come with me to see Cara," Paul insisted. "She has something important to tell you about."

"When? Now?"

"Yes. I've got my friend's car outside. I'll have you back by dinner."

"I can't," I protested. "Jobi would be afraid if I left, and . . ."

"Aunt Helen will be here, and it won't be for that long. Come on." He pulled me up.

"Wait—let me change clothes and put on makeup and . . ."

Paul smiled. "You don't need to do that for Cara."

172

39

SHE ASKED ME TO LIE on the floor. She put a pillow under my head. At first, I felt silly when she knelt behind me and began lightly to massage my temples. But when Cara started to speak in her gentle way, I relaxed.

"See yourself at the water's edge. Hear it lap at the shore. The tree you're sitting under . . . its leaves are rustling softly in the light breeze."

I was there. I experienced what Cara described to me. As she spoke, her whispered words seemed to cascade around me like colored butterflies. Her voice placed me on a soft cloud, and I rested. Every muscle in my body untensed for the first time in many months.

"Now I think we're ready to talk," said the tranquil woman, as she moved gracefully to sit cross-legged on the carpeting in front of me.

"I'm better," I said with amazement.

"I know," she replied with none. "I have a story to tell you. I think it will help."

And Cara, her ash blond hair pulled into a soft knot, her slender face serene, began to speak—forever changing my philosophy of life.

"When my daughter was two," said Cara, "she was burned horribly in a fire. Hospitalized, her chances were not good. Besides the danger from the burns, she refused to eat. Her body wasn't healing.

"One night I sat at her bedside and thought terrible thoughts. Hopeless thoughts. And then there was awakening.

173

A voice inside me said, 'Negative thoughts emit negative waves and produce negatives.' I pondered this strange idea, and then I understood.

"As my child settled into restless sleep, I saw her in my mind. I saw her wake, sit up, smile, and ask for food. I saw her eat and her burns begin to heal. I kept the image in my mind for a long time, sitting there by her bed.

"The next morning she fulfilled the dream. She ate for the first time in days, and I could almost sense the change occurring in her body. That night, once again I sat beside her as she slept. Now I saw her laughing and getting out of bed and walking about the room. The next morning, the image I created came to be. Each night after that, I used every ounce of my concentration to heal my child. And she is as you've seen her today; well, happy, and unscarred."

Cara's story had tremendous impact on me. My insides began to stir with excitement.

"You think I could do the same for Jobi." It was not really a question. I already knew I would.

Cara spoke softly but intently. "See her in a yellow light. It is Jobi's color of healing."

"Yellow. Of course." I knew her words almost before she said them. A strange warmth and feeling of awareness spread through me.

"See her as you wish her to be," said Cara.

"But I want her to dance." I faltered for a moment.

"Then see her dancing." Cara smiled. "And see her well."

I felt great strength flowing through me that evening. My body was relaxed, but my mind was taut and alert. I experienced a strong sense of mission.

While Jobi got ready for bed, I told my mother everything Cara had said. The intensity of my feelings transmitted itself to my mother, and I saw her eyes become bright with interest.

174

I explained to her what I planned to do that night, and she nodded her understanding.

"What if I did this . . . 'thinking' thing with you?" she asked.

I was surprised. I felt I should tell her what I was doing, but it hadn't occurred to me my mother would want to participate. Somehow I had never thought of her as the sort of person who could contemplate a rather spiritual experience. But then, once I wouldn't have believed this timid soul could help bandage an amputation wound or travel alone across the country.

"Yes! Good idea, Mother. The results would have to be twice as good if you do it with me." We hugged each other.

My mother and I tucked Jobi in bed together. My mother handed Mrs. Beasly to her, and I kissed her on the cheek.

"I'm sick of this place," Jobi frowned. " I want to go to sleep in my own bed."

"Soon, love. I promise." I kissed her again and turned off the light. The only illumination came faintly from the corridor. Laurel and the Petersons had gone home that morning, and Sarah had been moved temporarily to the Stanford Hospital for special treatment, so we had the room to ourselves.

Saying nothing, my mother and I each quietly pulled chairs on either side of Jobi's bed. We didn't have long to wait; the little girl was still weak from the drugs. She fell quickly asleep.

I don't know where my mother's mind took her that night, but the path of mine is unforgettable. I summoned a picture of Jobi in a long dress. She was dancing and a yellow glow surrounded her. Her skin shone with health and rosy color, and she laughed happily. Then the picture changed, and I saw Jobi's blood being taken the next morning; the slender line of crimson in the glass pipe. I watched the lab girl leave and even felt my restlessness as I waited for the time to pass until I could learn the results. And I watched myself walk

175

to the desk and ask Paula to call down to the lab for early results. I saw Paula dial and nod and look up at me. I saw her lips form the words and listened to the sound of her saying the words. "Two point two. Her white count is 2.2."

I sat without moving for over two hours, summoning the same scene to my mind over and over. At last I heard my mother sigh a little with exhaustion. I motioned her out of the room with me. Silently, we went to get some coffee. We sat in the kitchen facing each other.

"I never knew thinking could wear a person out." My mother smiled.

"I know just what you mean." I felt limp and drained of energy. But good. I felt good.

The next morning my eyes glued themselves to the lab girl. I watched her do exactly what I had pictured in my mind the night before. Jobi set up her usual howl and protest, unmollified even by making slides, but the finger stick was done anyway.

And then I sat in a chair and concentrated with all my might. I re-envisioned everything I wanted to happen—everything that must happen—again and again. At last the time came to act out my own role in the scene I created.

A flesh-and-blood me walked to Paula's desk and asked her to call the lab. Never for a moment while I waited for her to dial did I allow my mind to stop hearing her say, "Two point two." Dr. Short had said 2.0 was the white count necessary for Jobi to leave. So I provided a safe margin and called for 2.2.

Paula nodded and put down the receiver. She looked up at me. I stopped breathing. Had it worked? Could people actually use their minds and positive thoughts to change a blood count?

"Mrs. Halper, this is kind of strange," Paula said. "Jobi's white count has risen since yesterday from .9 to 2.2."

I couldn't move for a moment. I was frozen with surprise,

joy, relief, and even fear at what had happened. Then I let out a whoop of triumph.

"Thanks, Paula. I love you!" I shouted and ran to find my mother.

"We did it," I gasped. "We actually did it."

"What was the count?" she asked, tears beginning to drip down her cheeks.

"Two point two," I hollered, squeezing her. I whirled around as Jobi came into the room.

"Sunshine," I said, picking her up, her crutches falling to the ground. "We're going home."

PART THREE

40

HEIDI HAD MISSED ME a lot while I was gone. She told me recently about her bad feelings during my absence and even upon my return. She had tried to be closer to David, but his sadness was too much for her.

She remembers driving away from the hospital in California in the yellow "Gremil." She had felt all empty in her stomach watching Jobi and me grow smaller and smaller through the rear window as the car headed for the airport. She looked over at her father and was surprised to see tears in his eyes.

Heidi leaned over shyly and put her hand on David's arm. She and her father never kissed and hugged each other, so the touching came hard.

"Don't worry, Dad," she said, patting his arm a little. "I'll take care of you."

David had looked at her strangely and tried to wipe the tears from his eyes. But he didn't say anything.

His silence made Heidi feel embarrassed. She withdrew her hand and stared out the window. She wished she could make her father feel better, but she supposed only Jonathan could do that.

"That's how it is," she had thought bitterly. "Jonathan has Dad, Jobi has Mom, and I have no one."

It wasn't as though Heidi didn't feel awful about her sister's leg. She was very sorry for Jobi. But all those presents . . . and getting to stay in California with me. Sometimes, in a teeny tiny place within her, Heidi wished it had been she.

Often Heidi had felt guilty because her mind kept thinking things she didn't mean it to think; things like wondering what they did with Jobi's leg after it was cut off. Did they put it in a box and bury it in the backyard of the hospital? She and her friend Tracy had once buried a dead bird in Tracy's backyard. Or maybe the leg was put in a grocery bag and sent out with the garbage.

She didn't ask anyone about it. Even if she weren't too ashamed to let anyone know what she was thinking, whom could she ask? Jonathan was just a baby. Heidi wasn't sure if he really understood about Jobi at all. He still slept with a fuzzy piece of baby blanket.

And forget Dad, she had thought. Once home, her father's sadness often turned to anger. Heidi and David seemed to get into a fight if she so much as asked him what the temperature outside was. Of course, that was because usually the temperature was low, which caused him to tell her to wear her boots to school, a thing she hated to do.

She could have asked Grandma Edythe, who was staying with them while I was gone. But Heidi was afraid she'd get lecture number four hundred and sixty-seven. First Grandma Edythe would be shocked that Heidi could ask such a question, but she'd try not to show it. Then she was sure her grandmother would give her a long answer full of words she thought Heidi could understand. Grandma should only have known some of the words Heidi understood. And, one way or another, Heidi figured that Grandma Edythe would find a way to end with a discussion of Heidi's fights with her father, treatment of her little brother, and bad attitude in general. The lecture would end with, "Now dear, you feel free to come to me any time you have a question . . . even one like that."

While I was away, Heidi's home was a sad place, and she avoided it as much as possible. Her friend Lisa Plitman invited her over often and Heidi accepted eagerly. She loved being at the Plitmans'. Lisa's mother, who insisted on being called Charlene, took great interest in Heidi, making her feel

182

special. Charlene was among the few of her mother's friends who didn't remind Heidi she would have to give her mother a lot of help since she was the oldest. Charlene seemed to understand that Heidi also needed a lot of help at that time. After all, it was Heidi whose mother had left her for a month. It was Heidi who had to watch her younger sister become the center of attention and the recipient of gifts befitting a princess. What did Heidi receive? Hassles from her father and lectures from her grandmother. At the Plitmans', Heidi was treated as an honored guest.

The Plitmans were vegetarians—what Heidi's father called "health food nuts." But Heidi thought health foods tasted good and didn't mind the meatless dinners to which she was frequently invited. Of course, Heidi thought most food tasted good. That was another nice thing about Charlene Plitman; unlike David, Charlene never gave Heidi disapproving looks when she took second helpings. Heidi believed that her father thought everyone should be as thin as he and Jobi.

As my stay in California grew longer and longer, David became sadder and, to Heidi, seemed far away most of the time. The sadness in her home grew so strong, Heidi could hardly stand to be there. She began going over to the Plitmans' even when Lisa wasn't home. Charlene always welcomed her, and often they'd sit together on the Plitmans' big fluffy bed with the shades drawn and talk about Life, and Heidi's anger toward everyone in her family, an anger that directed itself mainly at me for being away and at Jobi for keeping me there.

When David brought Jobi and me home from the airport, Heidi had suddenly felt shy. At the time, when I tried to hug and kiss her, I didn't understand why she wiggled away. I thought it was because Heidi didn't like to be touched very much. It would be years before I found out about her anger.

She and Jobi didn't have a lot to say to each other. Heidi remembers feeling almost afraid of her sister, with her skinny arms that looked like sticks and her white, white skin. She wondered what they had done to her in that hospital in California.

But the worst was yet to come. One morning, Heidi heard Jobi crying in her bedroom. Heidi didn't see what Jobi had to cry about—sitting in that room full of giant stuffed animals and beautiful dolls. Heidi wanted so much to feel and hold the wonderful toys, but she wouldn't touch any of them.

She looked into her sister's pink bedroom. Jobi was sitting in her bed looking down at the pillow, and there was hair all over it—Jobi's hair. Heidi walked over to get a better look at this new phenomenon. She inspected Jobi's head . . . her hair didn't really look any different. It really wasn't such a big thing. So a little hair had fallen out. Jobi had plenty more.

"Hey," Heidi said to her sister, feeling a little sorry for her in spite of herself. "Want me to get that wig you brought home with you?"

I had explained to Heidi and Jonathan that Jobi might lose her hair from medicine and showed them the "just-in-case" wig. But Heidi's kind offer to fetch the wig had only brought higher pitched wailing from Jobi. With an exasperated sigh, Heidi went to get me.

I collaborated on the phone with my mother while Heidi was eating her breakfast. I was trying to keep my voice down because Jobi was on the couch in the family room and I didn't want to be overheard.

"No, I just can't bring myself to cut her hair short," I said into the receiver. "I know they recommended it, but not yet. Let's wait . . . maybe no more will fall out. What? Oh, say—that's a great idea, Mother."

Heidi had been bored with the one-sided conversation. She looked at her brother. If Jonathan was aware that a

184

minor catastrophe was occurring in the house, he gave no sign. Seeing me occupied, he stealthily shoved his hand to the bottom of the cereal box, trying to find the prize. I had made the rule that the lucky child whose bowl the prize landed in as the cereal was being poured got to keep it.

"Jonny, you cheater," Heidi hissed. "I'm telling."

Jonathan considered whether to risk the dire threat and decided against it. He withdrew his arm and with sticky fingers shoved the spilled cereal off the table and back into the box.

"Yech!" stated Heidi. "I'll never eat from that box of cereal again."

My mother came over after school with gum and candy for everyone. She wouldn't dare do that when David was home. He had absolutely forbidden candy and "junk" in the house. For all his mocking of the Plitmans' eating habits, something must have rubbed off on him. Since Jobi's illness, David had insisted I buy things such as raw sugar and whole wheat bread, and he began sprinkling wheat germ on all his food. But both Grandma Helen and Grandma Edythe sneaked junk food to their grandchildren whenever David's back was turned.

Today my mother had an extra gift for Jobi. Heidi sulked when she saw it, although she considered it a strange present. My mother brought Jobi a pink satin pillow case. She had heard somewhere that sleeping on a satin pillow case prevented hair loss.

It didn't. The next morning there was more hair on Jobi's pillow. My mother tried again to convince me to cut Jobi's hair. But I still couldn't bring myself to do it.

A few days later, Jobi came down the stairs on her crutches crying loudly. As she passed her sister, Heidi thought she looked really weird. Jobi's hair had matted together in sticky clumps all over her head. There were places where Heidi could see Jobi's head showing through the hair.

185

I took Jobi on my lap and hugged her until she stopped crying. Heidi later told me it looked as though I wanted to cry instead. She was right.

David came home and took in the situation.

"You should have cut it," he told me. Heidi didn't think that was the most helpful thing he could have said. She was right again.

Then I decided to phone Phil Kenton. Phil was a hairdresser, and David and I knew him well through mutual membership in a synagogue couples' club. Heidi heard me tell Phil what was happening and ask him what we should do.

Phil Kenton was at our house in ten minutes. He had brought a blue plastic cape with him, which he put around Jobi, and then sat her on two telephone books. With her matted hair, Jobi's head appeared small above the billowing cape. The hairdresser treated Jobi as though she were a grown-up woman.

Phil sat behind Jobi with scissors and a comb in his hand. He looked as though he didn't know how to start, and Heidi thought maybe he was going to get sick.

He lifted a long clump of matted hair and began to cut through it. The whole strand came off in his hand before the scissors closed. Heidi watched with amazement as a tear trickled down the man's cheek. The hairdresser was crying. He kept cutting, the hair mostly falling out as he touched it, and crying. I was watching and crying, although Heidi could see I was trying not to do it. Jobi started to cry, and Heidi had to brush some wetness away from her own face. It was everyone else's crying that made her feel so badly.

Finally Mr. Kenton had cut as much hair off as he could. There was only a thin layer left on Jobi's head, and Mr. Kenton tried to comb it so it would cover the worst of the bald spots. Jobi looked terrible, like Heidi's parakeet when it molted. But everyone told Jobi how cute her new haircut was. David tried to pay Mr. Kenton for coming to our house

186

and giving Jobi a haircut, but he acted insulted and wouldn't take anything.

As it turned out, the whole thing was a waste of time anyway. That night the rest of Jobi's hair fell out on the pink satin pillow case. All that was left on her head was a layer of fuzz, so pale it looked white. I took out the long blond wig and put it on Jobi's head before she got out of bed.

The wig was so big it wouldn't stay on straight. Heidi correctly guessed Jobi must have tried it on over her full head of hair when she bought it. Quickly I pulled a string inside which made the wig tighter. But Heidi thought it still looked terrible on Jobi.

Heidi was happy to find I agreed with her. I told her that Grandma and I were taking Jobi shopping for another wig that same day. But she was also irritated because she had to baby-sit with Jonathan while we were gone.

"You're a baby. I have to sit on you," she had taunted her brother after we left.

"Oh yeah?" he asked. "I'll tell."

"Then I'll tell about the cereal box."

"Then I'll tell about the Hydrox cookies you got under your bed."

"You monster!" she screeched and chased him around the kitchen table.

But Jon was saved from being sat upon. We wig shoppers had returned. Jobi was now wearing a short, darker blond wig with bangs. It looked better than the long one, but Heidi still thought Jobi looked awful. Heidi was disgusted by everyone's gathering around Jobi and telling her how cute she looked when she really looked rotten. Heidi went over to the Plitmans'.

41

OUR STAY AT HOME was all too brief. Less than three weeks later, Jobi and I flew back to California for her injection of Adriamycin. From now on I'd be on my own on these trips. Obviously, my mother couldn't continue to accompany me. I was determined to be a stronger, braver person and not give in to depression and self-pity again.

David and I had a warm reunion, and after my first night home, when he had made love to me with tenderness and passion, I silently whispered, "So there, Lois." The problems in my marriage, which were evident before Jobi's illness, still existed. But David and I needed each other too much to succumb to them at that time of crisis. I wouldn't allow myself even to contemplate the future, when shelved problems might return.

The only thing to mar our stay at home was the loss of Jobi's hair. It's hard to explain why, but Jobi's hair falling out was nearly as traumatic for both of us as her surgery. We adjusted in time, of course, and Jobi ended up with a large wig collection. I saw to it that she could wear her "hair" in pigtails, bangs, pulled back with barrettes, or nearly any other way she had ever worn her own hair. If she wasn't happy, at least she was content.

Oddly, I wasn't really sorry to be returning to Palo Alto. Adriamycin was the drug we had joined the protocol study to get. It was unobtainable anywhere in the United States except at Stanford Hospital for Children with Dr. Jordan Wilbur in charge. David and I both believed Adriamycin was the drug with the power to save Jobi.

Returning to the hospital was almost like coming home, albeit not exactly a cozy one. But at least it was familiar and no longer had the power to shock and horrify me as it had the first time I arrived.

Both Carl and Michael, two of the boys on the osteogenic sarcoma protocol study with Jobi, were at the hospital when we returned. Lois, Michael's mother, seemed more tense and brittle than ever, and I suspected Michael's medical reports were not good.

Another osteo patient arrived at the hospital the same day as we. Kevin was twelve years old, and his tumor had attacked his upper left arm. An experiment had been tried on Kevin. Rather than amputate his arm, the bone and muscle from the upper arm were removed, but the arm remained attached and the nerves intact. It was thought that while Kevin would not have much use of the arm, at least he would have one. As I watched him try to roughhouse with the other boys, his arm useless in a protective sling, I couldn't help thinking he'd have been better off with a prosthetic arm. Sadly, the experiment failed. A few months later the tumor returned, this time in Kevin's lower arm, and the limb had to be amputated after all.

Once again, on this trip, Lois was the bearer of information that shocked and frightened me.

"You haven't met Freddy Barton. You missed him; he left yesterday," Lois commented my first afternoon as we sat in the smoking lounge.

"No. Who's Freddy Barton?" I was looking out the long windows. One nice thing about being here, spring came to Palo Alto two months before Minneapolis. The grass was green, and flowers were already blooming.

"Freddy's the other boy on the protocol study. He had his leg amputated like the others."

"How's he doing on the drugs?"

"He's doing fine." Lois's eyes narrowed from the smoke. "It's his mother who's a mess."

"She's having trouble coping with Freddy's illness? I can understand that."

"I guess you could say that," Lois said slowly. "You see she's already lost another child to osteogenic sarcoma."

I looked at her in horror. She was almost smiling. I had the feeling Lois had actually enjoyed telling me the story.

"Two children in the same family with osteogenic sarcoma?" I breathed. My throat started to tighten and my hands felt clammy. "Are you trying to tell me osteo could be hereditary?"

"No one knows. But it seems possible, doesn't it?" Lois squashed out her cigarette. "See ya." She walked in the direction of her room.

I sat practically frozen to the spot. Heidi and Jonathan, I kept thinking. Could this happen to them too? Terror gripped me and I jumped up and nearly ran toward Dr. Wilbur's office. Something in my face must have told Wilbur's secretary it was not time to ask me to be seated and wait. She showed me right in to Dr. Wilbur's office.

I related Lois's story to him and my fear for my other children. He explained that the Barton family was a rare exception, and there was no reason to believe Heidi and Jonny were any more susceptible to cancer than other children. He calmed me down and reassured me, but I never completely rid myself of the nagging doubt that Lois had planted.

Before giving Adriamycin to Jobi, Dr. Wilbur ordered a series of nuclear X rays. These would be done at Stanford Hospital, and I tried not to feel panicky as we rode the van the few blocks between the two hospitals. Nuclear X rays . . . it sounded so frightening.

Jobi needed a bone scan, tomograms, and a skeletal survey. These were all special X rays to determine whether evidence of disease existed anywhere in her body. They were considered nuclear medicine because they utilized a safe but

190

nevertheless radioactive isotope to trace organs and bones. They would be taken of Jobi every three months for a year, and once a year for five years . . . if she had five years. The X rays weren't painful, but they were very time consuming. We were at Stanford all day, and amusing Jobi so she'd lie still wasn't easy. I've hated ticktacktoe ever since.

I was thankful that the X rays were all negative, and the next day Jobi was given Adriamycin. Dr. Short had a little bit of trouble with the I.V. needle. Jobi's veins were beginning to tire. I held her other hand tightly as the needle probed for a strong vein. She cried softly and I wished it were happening to me instead.

Once the vein was found, the administering of the Adriamycin took only a few minutes. I planned to leave the next day and return home until the next administration of the drug was due.

The power of Adriamycin to make Jobi sick made Cytoxan and methotrexate seem like aspirin. It took days until the violent nausea, cramps, and diarrhea receded. Jobi was very weak when we boarded the plane to go home. If it wasn't for the kindness of the Western Airline staff, our travel would have been impossible.

David had spoken to an official of the airline and explained our circumstance. He was assured Western would do everything it could to help. There was always a wheelchair waiting when we drove to the airport and when we deplaned. Whenever possible, we were given all three seats across so Jobi could lie down. And since we usually took the same flight in both directions, the flight attendants became like old friends, doing their utmost to make us comfortable. Once the pilot came and got Jobi and carried her to the cockpit, allowing her to ride there for a while.

Following the Adriamycin injection, Jobi was miserable during the three-hour plane ride home. While the worst of the nausea was over, she still felt ill and listless. But we both thought she'd be happier recovering at home.

191

Midflight, a man returning from the lavatory noticed Jobi lying with her head in my lap, her wig on lopsided. Her empty pant leg also must have been obvious. He returned to his seat and beckoned a flight attendant. Explaining he was a clown with the Shriners, he told her to let us know he'd be coming down the aisle in a few minutes to cheer up "the poor little girl." The flight attendant was aware Jobi wasn't feeling well and tried to dissuade the well-meaning Shriner, but to no avail.

She came to our seat to tell me about the "clown." Jobi looked up and said, "Tell him no, Mom. I feel icky. I don't want to talk."

"I tried to tell him, ma'am," the attendant replied in distress. "But . . . oh-oh, here he comes."

I shrugged my understanding that there was obviously no way to turn off the good-deeder, and she moved out of his way.

A jovial man with a huge belly, he knelt awkwardly in the aisle by our seat. Jobi sat up and tried to smile politely. The man seemed unaware that green was not her normal color. He had put on a big red clown nose and had a Punch puppet on his hand. Brushing away my attempt to explain how sick she was, he proceeded to use every trick at his command to get Jobi to laugh. He didn't realize she was using every trick of hers to keep from throwing up. Neither one of their tricks worked.

"The bag, Mom, the bag," Jobi gasped, covering her mouth with her hands. As she used the bag noisily, our friend the clown turned pale, removed his nose, and beat a hasty retreat back down the aisle. But that's show business.

42

DR. WILBUR DECIDED there was no reason Jobi couldn't take her seven days of Cytoxan at home, with Dr. McMillan standing by in case of trouble. Jobi would have her monthly chest X ray at the Suburban Medical Clinic, where McMillan was on staff, as well as blood tests every week.

As usual, it was the blood test that caused all the trouble, but now of a different sort. I took Jobi to the clinic where Dr. McMillan checked her over and pronounced her fit. Needing lab reports for comparative study after the Cytoxan would be administered, he sent us upstairs for her chest X ray and blood work. The chest film was quickly taken, and as before, I looked at it carefully. But I still had no idea what to look for. Sighing, I put the X ray film back in the envelope; I'd have to wait until tomorrow.

I led Jobi down the hall to where a sign said Lab. I handed the blood work order to a young technician who asked Jobi to have a seat on a chair in the cluttered, but sterile-looking room. Jobi began to become agitated as usual and grabbed for my hand. I tried to talk her into calmness, reminding her that a finger stick takes less than a second.

As I spoke, I realized the technician was wrapping elastic around Jobi's left arm.

"What are you doing?" I asked her.

"Applying pressure so the vein stands out better," she explained politely. "That makes it easier to draw the blood."

"That's not what I mean," I interrupted her. "Why are you drawing blood from her arm. Just prick her finger."

The young woman looked up at me, startled.

"The kind of tests your doctor ordered can't be done with a finger prick," she said carefully, as if explaining to a child.

"May I see the orders?" I was even amazing myself.

Her face hardened and she handed me the order sheet. I looked it over quickly. The tests ordered were the identical ones done every morning in Palo Alto . . . with a finger stick.

"These tests are done at Stanford Hospital for Children on a daily basis with a finger stick," I said firmly.

"Well here, they're done by drawing blood from the arm," she said pointedly, tightening the band on Jobi's arm.

"Look, these kids have needles in their veins all the time. We don't want to use her veins except for the drugs," I appealed to her, hoping she'd soften.

"Ma'am, I'm telling you, I can't get enough blood with a finger stick for these tests. We have our own way of doing things here. Period."

Now I was angry. This was just a power struggle with Jobi's poor veins being the prize. I looked around the room and my eyes rested on what I'd been seeking. There on a table stood a Coulter Counter.

"You see that little machine over there, dear?" I said sweetly to the scowling lab technician. "That is a Coulter Counter. It's a wonderful invention." I raised my voice. "It can perform dozens of tests from just a few drops of blood!"

She looked at me furiously. Apparently I was not supposed to be so knowledgeable. Jobi, in the meantime, had forgotten it was her blood being fought over. She was having a wonderful time listening to the adults fight—she tried to cover up a grin.

"I'm very sorry," the lab technician said through tight lips. "I can do this blood work only by drawing blood from the patient's arm."

"That isn't true," I told her coldly. "But in that case, we're leaving. Come on, Jobi."

"Wait—you can't do that." The girl was confused now.

194

I could see she wondered if she would end up in trouble over the entire affair.

"Sure I can," I said cheerfully, handing Jobi her crutches. "Take the blood with a finger stick or we're leaving."

"I—I'll call your doctor," she said and rapidly disappeared into another room. I could hear the low angry murmur of her voice on the phone.

She came back into the room. "I'll do the finger stick," she said grimly.

Jobi grinned at me triumphantly until she realized she still had to have her finger pricked with a needle. The grin left and she began her usual protest. That never changed, but no one ever again tried to draw blood from her arm at the Suburban Medical Clinic.

43

JOBI'S TWO BEST FRIENDS during her year of chemotherapy were Dana Plitman and Judy Sher. Many other children visited and helped her, but these two girls were her ever-present companions. Their dedication amazed me, and I wondered at the maturity of these nine-year-old children in dealing with life-and-death matters. I also pondered at their motives. . . . What prompted the two little girls to sacrifice so much of their time and spend it in the often unpleasant company of a sick child?

As teenagers, both Dana and Judy related to me their thoughts and feelings during the time of Jobi's illness. Both girls remember events with startling clarity.

Dana Plitman held Jobi's hand during the drive to the Suburban Medical Clinic. Dana knew her friend was very upset about the shot she would receive today. She knew because while they were still back in Jobi's bedroom, Jobi had cried.

"I'm scared, Dana," Jobi had whimpered. "I can't do it. . . . It hurts too much. I couldn't even stand the blood test I had yesterday."

Dana had swallowed and looked away from Jobi's brimming eyes. Dana didn't know what to say. She was scared to death of shots herself. But her mother had told her Jobi might die if she didn't get the shots.

Dana remembered the first time her mother had told her about her distant cousin, Jobi Halper, last fall. Her mother said Jobi, a year younger than nine-year-old Dana, was very sick. Dana knew Heidi Halper very well because Heidi and Dana's sister Lisa were friends. But she and Jobi were in different grades at school and knew each other only to greet in passing.

As gently as possible, Dana's mother had told her that Jobi had cancer and her leg had been amputated. Quick tears of sympathy had sprung to Dana's dark eyes. Her mother suggested perhaps Dana should go to visit the sick child and offer to be of help. Dana thought her mother's idea was a good one and ran quickly to fetch her coat.

About to leave and walk the few blocks between the Plitman and Halper homes, Dana had an idea. Excitedly, she ran to the kitchen and found a plastic bag. She brought it to the enormous bedroom-playroom she shared with her two sisters and half-filled the bag with water from her aquarium. She took a small net down from the shelf and scooped up her favorite fish, a handsome blue Beta who wiggled in protest. Dana flopped him into the bag of water and twisted the top tightly. Carefully she walked to the front door carrying the fish away from her body. Her mother came into the foyer and smiled when she saw the Beta. Dana was aware her mother knew the fish was among Dana's prized possessions.

196

"It's a little chilly out today for fish," said Dana's mother, putting on her coat. I'll drive you two over to the Halpers'."

Judy Sher and Jobi Halper had been friends since first grade—a long time in the life span of an eight-year-old. But of all the experiences they had shared, Judy would forever remember the November day she had had the fight with a boy in her class at school. Judy and Jobi were standing on the playground, and Judy and the boy were exchanging taunts. The boy was getting angrier and angrier with Judy. He threatened to get even. Judy laughed and ran behind her friend Jobi just as the boy drew back his leg to kick her. The kick landed solidly and with a sickening thud on Jobi's left leg, just below the knee. Jobi wailed loudly from both pain and injustice, and the boy ran away.

Time passed and Jobi's leg kept hurting. Then one day Judy and her friend, Sue Brennon, came to call for Jobi so the three girls could walk to school together as usual. But Jobi's mother told them Jobi's leg hurt her so much she couldn't go to school.

Judy and Sue were puzzled that their friend's leg should hurt for such a long time. They wondered if maybe Jobi just wanted to "skip school."

The next day Judy's mother told her they were going over to Sue Brennon's house for a few minutes. The Brennons', Shers', and Halpers' backyards all touched, so it took only a short time to walk between the houses. Judy wondered why her mother was taking her over to the Brennons'. She had never done anything like that before.

When they arrived, Mrs. Brennon asked Judy and her mother to sit down at the kitchen table with Sue. She poured coffee for Mrs. Sher and set out a plate of cookies. Mrs. Sher didn't drink the coffee, and the room was very quiet. Judy was beginning to feel nervous and she looked questioningly at Sue. But Sue raised her eyebrows and shrugged a little— she didn't know what this strange meeting was about either.

Mrs. Brennon sat down at the table and said, "We have something sad to tell you. Our little friend Jobi is very sick and has to have an operation."

Judy could hardly believe it . . . Jobi, sick enough to need an operation.

"You know how her leg's been sore?" Mrs. Brennon continued. The two little girls nodded solemnly. "Well, they found out there's a tumor in her leg . . . cancer . . ."

Mrs. Brennon stopped and blew her nose. Mrs. Sher opened her purse and found a handkerchief to wipe her eyes. Judy felt her stomach lurch. What was going on? It couldn't be Jobi they were talking about.

"They have to . . . to amputate her leg so she can get well." Mrs. Brennon could hold back her tears no longer. She cried harshly, and Mrs. Sher buried her face in her hands. Judy and Sue began to cry as well. Judy wasn't even sure she understood what was happening. Amputate . . . what did it mean? When her mother explained it to her later, she went into her room and cried and cried.

Dana Plitman and Judy Sher didn't know each other very well, but they both happened to choose the same day and moment to visit Jobi, who had recently arrived home from the hospital.

Judy, arms laden with cookies, a stuffed animal, and a coloring book, and Dana, gingerly carrying the blue Beta, arrived at the same time and walked up the steps in front of the Halpers' brick and stucco home. They smiled warily at each other, and Dana, the only one who could free a hand, rang the door bell.

As they waited for the door to be opened, both girls were nervous. Dana suddenly wondered what she would say to a sick person she scarcely knew. Judy was even more afraid. What would her friend Jobi look like now . . . and how did you talk to someone with one leg?

198

Both girls remember that I had greeted them and led them to the family room where Jobi was lying on the couch. She was wearing a long pink nightgown and looked no different than she had ever looked . . . except she was moaning a little.

"Hi Jobi—how are you?" asked Judy cheerfully, relieved Jobi didn't look like a monster. Dana stood shyly back, still clutching the bag with the fish.

"Hi," Jobi said weakly. "Oh . . . my toes . . . I feel my toes curling the wrong way." Her face twisted in pain. Judy didn't know what Jobi was talking about.

"Jobi gets phantom pains," I had explained. "She feels pain in the missing leg." The girls watched me as I took a small pill from a bottle on the TV tray next to Jobi. I had two spoons with me, and I used one spoon to crush the pill in the other spoon. Then I mixed some grape jelly into the powdered pill, explaining, "Jobi can't swallow pills, so she has to 'eat' her pain medication."

Dana grimaced watching Jobi try to swallow the powdered pill mixed with jelly. She had thought how awful it must taste. Just as Jobi finished with a shudder, Dana remembered the Beta in her hands.

"Here—this is for you," Dana beamed, her white teeth flashing against her olive skin.

Jobi sat up and grinned when she saw the beautiful blue fish swimming in the plastic bag.

"Hey—neat! Thanks, Dana."

Judy's naturally ruddy cheeks flamed. The coloring books and crayons, gifts to Jobi, had brought only a wan smile. Two enemies, Judy Sher and Dana Plitman, were born at that moment.

As the weeks passed, the two girls both nurtured a growing devotion to Jobi and an equally burgeoning dislike for each other. They avoided each other as much as possible, each staking out her own territory.

Judy rode in the car with Jobi each morning when I drove her to school. The girls were in the same class, and through the day, Judy was Jobi's other leg, carrying books for her, pushing doors open. Judy stayed in the schoolroom with her during lunch so Jobi wouldn't have to maneuver down the two flights of stairs to the lunch room. Judy sometimes felt resentful when one of the men teachers decided to carry Jobi down the stairs so she could eat lunch with the other children.

Dana took the night shift. Each day after school, Dana came to visit Jobi and play nurse. She learned how to wrap the Ace bandage around Jobi's stump and massage it when the phantom pains came. She coaxed her friend into doing the exercises the doctor had prescribed, and Dana was allowed to crush Jobi's pills and mix them with jelly. She often stayed for dinner, secretly relishing the meat-filled meals the Halpers enjoyed. She didn't tell her vegetarian parents how much she really liked meat. But she did tell her mother of her mixed emotions when she left Jobi each night . . . the sadness over her friend's illness mingled with the fulfillment of having been of help.

Both Dana and Judy were ferociously protective of Jobi. Both were prone to fly into defensive rages if any schoolchildren were overheard whispering about Jobi. One day after Jobi's hair had fallen out, Judy saw a man staring openly at Jobi. The children had been playing hopscotch, a game at which Jobi excelled, and her wig was askew.

"Take a picture," Judy shrieked angrily at the man. "It lasts longer!"

Dana's preoccupation with Jobi became almost an obsession. She thought about Jobi all the time. When she woke in the middle of the night needing to use the bathroom, she would hurry down the darkened hallway thinking, "If I were Jobi, first I'd have to find my crutches or I'd have to hop." Once she tried to hop down the hall, but she fell. When she went ice-skating that winter, she thought about Jobi, and gladness for her own health mingled with pity for her friend's lack of it. She cried, and the Minnesota wind caused the droplets to freeze on her cheeks.

Judy and Dana took turns accompanying Jobi to the doctor's office for X rays or blood tests or checkups. But it happened to be Dana who was with her when Jobi received her drug injection at the Suburban Medical Clinic. The preceding treatments had been done in California; this would be the first at home.

Comforting Jobi as best she could while they rode to the appointment, Dana was almost as frightened as Jobi. Dana was allowed to push Jobi into the medical center in a wheelchair, and when we were shown into the examining room where Dr. McMillan would see Jobi, I kissed and hugged Dana. Then I sat down next to Jobi and held her hand. Dana stood near her.

Dr. McMillan and his nurse, Jane, came breezily into the room. He joked with us and surprisingly remembered Dana's name from the last time she had been there with Jobi for her chest X ray. Seating himself in front of Jobi, he spoke reassuringly to her and selected a needle from the tray Jane held for him. He took Jobi's left hand and looked for a suitable vein. Each time he tried to insert the needle, Jobi pulled her hand away from him, her eyes wide with terror.

Dr. McMillan continued talking to Jobi gently but firmly, trying again and again to put the needle into her vein. I bent down and whispered something into Jobi's ear. Dana couldn't hear exactly what I said, but she thought it sounded like "deep . . . breaths . . . see yourself by a lake. . . ."

Finally Jobi held still and Dr. McMillan put the needle into her vein. Dana instinctively turned away as Jobi cried out, but something made her turn back to watch. Perhaps if she shared what was happening to Jobi, she could somehow make it easier for her friend to bear. She watched intently as the nurse placed a board under Jobi's arm to keep it still and Dr. McMillan injected two tubes of medicine into the needle.

Jobi became ill in the car on the way home, and Dana held the blue plastic bowl the nurse had given Jobi to use "just in case." I had smiled my appreciation to Dana, maneuvering my car through heavy Highway 100 traffic. As Jobi retched, Dana felt sick herself. But she steeled herself, thinking, "If this were happening to me, I'd want my friend to be there."

44

JOBI'S CHEST X RAYS continued to be clear. The waits for X rays to be read never shortened, and my breathless anxiety caused by the waiting never lessened. But each month that passed brought more hope.

David and I had been told that Jobi's ten percent chance of living would increase if the tumor did not appear in her lungs within the first six months. A year without disease would be cause for real hope, but she would not be considered completely out of danger for five years after the onset of the tumor.

Our third trip to Palo Alto in the spring of the year was relatively free of anxiety. Nearly six months had passed since Jobi's surgery, and I no longer dreamed that Jobi disappeared in the night.

Jobi was glum on the plane. The novelty of travel had waned, and she was tired of leaving her friends and home. And, of course, as her veins became weaker and more diffi-

202

cult to inject, her fear of the needles grew. But her natural high spirits prevailed, and soon a flight attendant had her giggling over some animals he made for her out of balloons.

I was almost relieved to find Lois had taken Michael home the day before I arrived at Stanford Hospital for Children. I was full of compassion for Lois and her son, whose lung tumor, I learned, was not responding to treatment, but I didn't feel up to Lois's bitter cynicism on this trip.

I greeted Emily Denton with mixed emotions. I was delighted to see the congenial southern woman, but her presence meant Robbie's brief remission from leukemia was over.

Emily filled me in on the arrival of a new patient, a tiny three-year-old boy from Malaysia who suffered the same malady as little Amy Peterson. The child had lost one eye to cancer and now because of unsuccessful surgery at home, another tumor had formed behind his other eye. The people in his small Malaysian village had collected money to send the boy to the United States for treatment when local doctors had pronounced him incurable. Little "Mo," as we called him, his real name being almost unpronounceable, was accompanied by his grandfather. The pair could speak no English, and while we all tried to be as friendly as possible, the language barrier was formidable.

"Dr. Wilbur has great hope for the li'l tyke," Emily told me. I didn't ask her if there was hope for her son, Robbie, as well. Somehow I knew by looking behind her warm smile, there was little. I fought the unspoken reminder that all Dr. Wilbur's patients were here because they had been given up as hopeless cases somewhere else.

Jobi received her methotrexate injection the next morning. It took several hours to drip into her arm, and we ticktack-toed it until I thought I'd scream if I saw another X. She was sick all night and threw a tantrum when the nurse came to inject the rescue medication into the tubing that led to the needle already in her vein.

"It's cold and it will hurt," Jobi screamed. "Stop! Don't do it!"

The young nurse looked at me knowingly and winked her reassurance that she could handle the situation.

"I've got an idea, Jobi," said the nurse. "Someone told me you want to be a doctor when you grow up . . . well, it's time you got a little practice."

Jobi stopped crying and looked at her with sudden interest.

"Here's what we'll do," the young woman said seriously. "I'll get the needle into the tube, and you push the medicine in yourself."

Jobi thought this over and decided it was a wonderful idea. Somehow when Jobi pushed the plunger on the needle herself, the medicine didn't feel as cold and didn't hurt . . . she injected her own rescue every time after that night.

I had just finished taking a morning shower and dressing when Paula, the head nurse, came to find me. Jobi had been wheeled to the classroom where the teacher was waiting to help her with the homework we had brought with us from Minneapolis.

"Sharon, there's someone here to see you," called Paula through the door of the huge community women's room. I wondered if it could be Paul. It didn't seem likely; he had met us at the airport and driven us to the hospital only two days before. It was a long drive to make again so soon.

The nurse entered the room as I quickly combed out my hair. "She's waiting in the kitchen."

"All right, thanks, Paula." She . . . I couldn't think of any "she" who would visit me. My sister-in-law, the capricious Bobby Sue, had taken off for parts unknown, and I didn't know anyone else in the area.

Seated on one of the hardback chairs lining the wall in the kitchen was a small plump woman about my own age.

She had thick shiny dark hair hanging loose to her shoulders and black horn-rimmed glasses that were falling off her very small nose. She looked a little nervous and uncomfortable, and she restlessly fingered a pile of what were clearly presents in her lap.

When I entered the room, she stood up, the presents falling to the floor.

"Hello," I said, trying to avoid laughing at her attempt to smile, introduce herself, and retrieve her packages all in the same motion.

"Hi. Are you Sharon? I'm Joan Cohen. I'm really glad to meet you." The words came tumbling in almost one breath. Joan grinned broadly and stuck out her hand to shake hands with me and managed to drop all the packages again.

"Oh, forget it," she said with exasperation and sat back in a chair. The presents remained on the floor where they had dropped. "Where's Jo Beth?"

"Uh . . . she's in the classroom." I wasn't sure how to respond to this amusing, but unusual woman.

"They have school here for the kids? Oh—that's wonder-ful!"

"Yes, it is, but . . ."

"Oh, I'm sorry. You don't even know me and here I'm running off without explaining."

I smiled my acceptance of this apology. I decided Joan Cohen was a delightful person, if a bit unconventional.

"You know Jerry and Arlene Fingerman, right?" Joan continued.

"Why yes—Arlene's father and my father are business partners. We were very good friends in school, but we hardly see each other anymore."

"Well, last winter Gordon and I—Gordon's my husband —we met the Fingermans on a vacation in Mexico. We stayed at Las Breesas. Have you ever been there? Such a

205

paradise," she sighed dramatically, then continued without waiting for my reply. "Arlene and Jerry are such nice people. We had a wonderful time with them.

"So Arlene called us when she found out you were coming to Palo Alto and told us all about you and Jo Beth. She said you didn't have any family or friends here, so we took a family vote and decided to be it."

"Be it?" I had trouble following this rapid torrent of words, but the overall gist made me warm to this woman even more.

"Be your family and friends," Joan smiled happily. "The Cohens are adopting you."

Before I could utter a word, she picked up the presents and put them in my lap. "These are for you and Jo Beth."

"Joan—thank you. I don't know what to say."

"Don't worry. According to Gordon, no one ever gets to say anything around me anyway."

We both laughed, and impulsively, I leaned over and kissed Joan Cohen's rosy cheek. She looked startled, then pleased. Her eyes misted over a little.

"I'm really so glad to meet you," she said softly, covering my hands with hers. "We want to do anything we can to help."

"This is so nice of you, Joan. We don't know anyone here except my cousin who visits from San Francisco sometimes. Jobi and I get a little lonesome for home. . . ."

"We'll be home. You call her Jobi? Listen, will they let you take her out of here for a while?"

"Yes. I don't know," I tried to answer both questions at once. "Right now she has to be hooked up to an I.V. unit every few hours, but they use a heparin lock so she doesn't have to lug around all that paraphernalia every minute."

"I don't know what all that means. Was it a yes or a no?"

I laughed and explained to Joan about the high-dose

methotrexate Jobi had received and the rescues now being administered every three hours.

Joan looked satisfied. "Well, if she has this rescue stuff, and we come and get you right away, we can keep you for three hours, right?" She didn't allow me to answer. "Great. You tell me what time, and Gordon will come back and get you. You and Jo Beth, I mean Jobi, are having dinner at our house tonight. Does Jobi like blintzes?"

"Joan, that's so sweet of you. But it's really more complicated than you think. She has to drink several glasses of liquid during the three hours in between, and getting her to do it is like pulling teeth. Oh—and also we have to measure every time she voids; they're very insistent about that. She could even get nauseated and be sick! It's just too enormous an imposition to put on anyone. But thank . . ."

"Does she like blintzes?" She acted as though I hadn't spoken. "I make the best cheese blintzes you ever tasted."

"Yes, she usually does. But Joan, she hardly eats anything right now."

"Wait till she meets Josh and Rachel and Amy and Ishmael and Jordy and all the rest. Rachel's just Jobi's age. Eight—right?"

"Yes, she'll be nine in April. Are all those your children?"

"No, some of them are animals. But then sometimes the children are animals, so it's hard to tell. Now, here's my phone number. I'm going shopping now, but you call me later and tell me what time Gordon should pick you up. You'll know who he is when he arrives—he's six feet tall, he wears glasses, and he's very distinguished-looking; like a psychiatrist, because that's what he is."

I tried to protest further as I accompanied Joan to the door, but she brushed over my attempts.

I had enjoyed meeting Joan but remained skeptical about the proposed visit to her home. After all, these were perfect strangers. How could I just get in a car with a strange man and have dinner with people I didn't know?"

As I gave myself reasons for refusing the invitation, I found myself walking back to the nursing station.

"Uh—Paula, I don't suppose I could take Jobi out of the hospital for a few hours tonight?"

"I don't see why not. I'll double-check with Dr. Wilbur, but as long as you get her back in time for the next Leucovorin, there's no problem."

Suddenly a feeling of happiness flooded over me. Of course I would take Jobi to visit the Cohens. It would be good for both of us to get away from the hospital for a while, and I wanted Jobi to laugh and play with children who weren't sick. Now if only Jobi herself wouldn't feel too sick to go.

45

MIRACULOUSLY, MY PALE DAUGHTER was not experiencing nausea that evening. I had called Joan and told her Jobi would receive her medication at five and wouldn't have to return to the hospital until eight. Doctor Wilbur said we had a half-hour leeway, and eight-thirty would be an equally acceptable return time.

Joan seemed very pleased and told me Gordon would be there at five-fifteen. I heard dogs barking and children laughing in the background. Then a vacuum cleaner sounded and drowned out the other voices.

"Greta!" Joan shrieked. "I can't hear!" The vacuum noise ceased. "That's my cleaning lady. She doesn't clean anything, but I like her because she makes neat piles."

I laughed with Joan, thinking, here is a girl after my own heart.

I told Jobi all about my visit from Joan Cohen, and by the time Gordon came for us, she was beside herself with excitement.

"They have a bunch of animals, Mom?"

"Yes, yes, it sounded like a whole zoo."

"Oh good! And Rachel's my age?"

"Yes, love. I'm sure we'll have a wonderful time. But remember, you promised to keep drinking your liquids there—otherwise we can't go."

"I will. I promise."

I helped her dress in her favorite outfit—pink flare-leg cotton pants, a pink blouse, and a pink, white, and orchid smock. She had worn the outfit all over Disneyland and put it on whenever she considered the occasion special.

We went to the side door of the hospital to wait for Gordon Cohen's arrival. Jobi's usually pale cheeks wore bright splotches of pink from excitement. She was in her wheelchair—she couldn't manage crutches while the needle remained in her hand with its heparin solution preventing the vein from closing. But if it were possible to be jumping up and down in a wheelchair, that is what Jobi was doing.

Gordon Cohen got out of his car and entered the building. He was exactly as Joan had described him, with the addition of a warm smile and twinkling eyes.

"Hi Jobi!" he said and kissed her cheek. "Sharon, I'm Gordon Cohen." And much to my surprise, he kissed me too. "Is everybody ready?"

I started to push the wheelchair to the door when Gordon said, "What do we need that for?"

"Jobi can't use her crutches with the needle in her arm," I explained.

"Is that all?" he scoffed. And to Jobi's delight, he scooped her up and carried her piggyback out the door, prancing and making horse noises.

I don't know why I felt tears slide down my cheeks. It just felt so good to find a friend.

The Cohens had a sprawling California rambler decorated in cluttered comfort. It looked much what mine might have looked like if David hadn't lived there with me, demanding neatness. I loved it.

Joan and Gordon's children seemed like family immediately. Their son Josh, about eleven, was a California boy with golden skin and golden curly hair. He was friendly and bright, and when I later learned he had made several commercials, I was hardly surprised.

Rachel, age eight, was a replica of her mother, complete with glasses falling off the end of a tiny nose. She and Jobi looked at each other shyly for a moment when they met. Two minutes later, Rachel demanded that Gordon carry Jobi to her bedroom so she could "play Barbie dolls with my new best friend."

Little Amy was an enchanting four-year-old who emitted a steady monologue of questions without pausing for answers. Two collies, three cats, two guinea pigs, an undisclosed number of rabbits in an outside hutch, and a few caged creatures I didn't fully investigate made up the rest of the Cohen family.

Gordon, Joan, and I sat in the living room getting acquainted for a while before dinner. They seemed sincerely interested in hearing about the rest of my family and a more detailed background on Jobi. They were so easy to talk to, I found myself unburdening myself more fully than I had to anyone else. They both appeared deeply moved as I described our discovery of Jobi's illness and the subsequent events that led us to Palo Alto.

"There's no question in my mind that Jobi is going to be just fine," stated Joan with firm conviction. Gordon agreed.

I smiled, grateful for their sincere reassurance, and was about to tell them about Paul and Wang when I remembered

Jobi had had nothing to drink for forty-five minutes. She was supposed to consume three eight-ounce glasses of liquid during the three-hour interval between medications. She never wanted to drink anything, and it usually took her nearly an hour to get one glass down.

"Do you have some kind of juice I could give Jobi to drink?" I asked, praying they would have one of the few kinds she would drink.

"Of course," laughed Joan. "We're all prepared."

"I'll go get Jobi so she can choose what she likes," said Gordon, getting to his feet. But before he could take a step we heard the thump thump thump that meant Jobi was managing on her own steam. The Cohens watched with amazement as Jobi hopped agilely into the room, giggling, followed by a much impressed Rachel.

I laughed. "Jobi can hop faster than most people can walk."

Joan recovered her composure. "Jobi, come with me into the kitchen, and I'll let you pick something to drink."

Gordon began to move toward the chair where Jobi had flopped. I saw the flash of mischief in her eye. Just as he reached to lift her, she dodged and jumped up. With a snicker, she hopped away after Joan. Rachel followed her reverently.

Gordon sat back in his armchair, shaking his head. "Incredible," he chuckled, filling a pipe. "Sharon, you know I'm a psychiatrist, but what you may not know is that I specialize in children."

"No, Joan didn't mention that."

"Frankly, I was prepared to offer my services to you and Jobi. I was sure she'd be having some emotional difficulties after the ordeal she's been through. But the child I met here this evening is bright, happy, and seems completely well adjusted. I'm amazed."

I smiled, inwardly wondering if he realized the mother might be suffering from the ordeal more than the child. But I just said, "I know what you mean. I keep waiting for her to react—cry, scream, carry on. But she doesn't. Oh, she might stage a protest against blood tests or swallowing pills, but basically, she seems undisturbed about the whole thing. I don't know whether to be glad or worried."

Gordon considered. "Well, for the moment, I think you should just wait. If counseling seems needed later, fine. For now, just . . ."

"Go with the flow?" He chuckled at my use of popular teenage vernacular and nodded. We heard Jobi and Rachel laughing in the kitchen, and I excused myself to go and see what new mischief my impish daughter was perpetrating.

The kitchen was a bedlam of pots and pans on the stove, groceries obviously still not put away since Joan's shopping trip, and general dinner preparation litter. I could sense the room was perfectly clean, but neatness definitely did not count.

Jobi was seated at the table across from Rachel and Amy, playing eeny meeny miney moe with at least a dozen cans and bottles of assorted beverages.

"My heavens—what's going on?" I asked.

"I told you we were prepared," beamed Joan. "I figured she'd have to like something we bought."

"I should hope so," I laughed.

Jobi made her decision, some cranberry-apple juice, and I reminded her she couldn't dawdle over it. Little Amy, who had followed her sister and Jobi into the kitchen earlier, had been strangely quiet since she had seen Jobi hopping.

I assumed Joan had told all three children about Jobi's condition, but now Amy said, "How come you don't got a leg?"

Joan froze, and I opened my mouth to make a diplomatic explanation, when Jobi calmly replied, "I lost it."

Amy looked solemn for a minute, then brightened. "Well, did ya try looking for it?"

Joan touched my arm; I looked at her. We didn't know whether to laugh or cry.

212

But Jobi did. She laughed. "No Amy, I didn't lose it like that."

Amy looked at her sternly. "Did you go in the street when your mother told you not to?"

Now Joan and I had to laugh. But we turned our faces to conceal our amusement because the discussion was still going on.

"You're just a little kid, Amy, so you don't understand," said Jobi with a superior air. "A boy kicked me and I got a tumor in my leg and the doctor had to take it away so I wouldn't get any more tumors."

As simple as that.

46

THE DAY AFTER Jobi and I were "adopted" by the Cohens, Dr. Wilbur came to talk with me. I was always pleased to see the tall, handsome Jordan Wilbur. His very presence seemed to strengthen my belief in Jobi's recovery.

"Has anything been done about a prosthesis for Jobi?" he asked after greeting me.

"Prosthesis?" I had never heard the term before.

"That means artificial limb," he explained. "Has she been fitted for one at home?"

"Why no—none of our doctors have said anything about it. I assumed it was too early."

Dr. Wilbur frowned. "It's not too early at all. I think we should take care of it immediately."

"All right."

"When were you planning to leave for home?" the doctor asked thoughtfully.

"Tomorrow," I answered firmly.

"I better get right on it." He beamed and rose to leave.

"You mean you're going to have a leg made for her before tomorrow?" I asked in surprise.

"Not quite . . . but close." I heard him chuckle as he walked down the hall with long strides, white coat flapping.

That afternoon Paula told me I was to take Jobi to a certain room in the basement of the hospital where an orthopedic doctor was waiting to see us. I realized the appointment had something to do with Jobi's prosthesis, but I was a little apprehensive as I pushed her wheelchair into the elevator. Dr. Pelletier was the only orthopedic doctor I had ever met, and I had hoped he'd be the last.

"Where're we going, Mom?" Jobi was annoyed. I had pulled her away from a game with Jo Anna Painter, who had arrived that morning.

"I think they're going to make you an artificial leg— they call it a prosthesis."

"Will it hurt?"

"Oh no—I'm sure there's nothing painful about it." I silently prayed I was right. Jobi was becoming more and more sensitive to pain. She couldn't seem to tolerate the slightest physical discomfort, crying even for so small a sensation as feeling too warm. This mysterious and frequent feeling of being hot bothered some of the other chemotherapy patients too, but no one seemed afflicted by it as much as Jobi.

Dr. Wilbur was waiting for us when we got off the elevator. He took us to a large room filled with odd-looking equipment and introduced us to Dr. Grant. Jobi's eyes were very large as she surveyed the room, and she looked warily at the white-streaked apron worn by Dr. Grant.

The orthopedist was nothing like the infamous Pelletier. A stockily built man, Dr. Grant was jovial and pleasant, putting us both at our ease.

214

"We're going to make a new leg for you, honey," he said cheerfully to Jobi.

"Will it look just like my old one?" she asked.

"As close as we can get it," he promised.

Explaining as he did it, Dr. Grant carefully measured Jobi's stump.

"Your orthopedist did an excellent piece of surgery here," he commented. You're very lucky. When the amputation is not done perfectly, the fitting of a prosthesis becomes a difficult job . . . sometimes impossible. But we shouldn't have any trouble with Jobi's fitting."

Measuring complete, Dr. Grant had Jobi balance on her leg and rest her stump in a metal clamp on a stand. Next, strips of gauze soaked in what appeared to be liquid plaster were wrapped around and around the stump. The gauze dried and the resulting cast, a mold of her stump, was removed.

"We'll use this to make you a socket," Dr. Grant said to Jobi, who was still giggling because he had made pen notations all over her stump before the casting, and they hadn't rubbed off yet.

"What does that mean . . . socket?" I wondered out loud.

"The socket is the most important part of the prosthesis—the part the stump rests in," Dr. Grant explained.

"The person who makes it has to be part skilled craftsman, part artist," interjected Dr. Wilbur, who had surprised me by staying to watch the procedure.

"Will you be making the limb, Dr. Grant?" I asked.

"Oh no—I'm no artist." He winked at Dr. Wilbur. "The prosthesis will be made from this cast by a certified prosthetist . . . a person trained in the making and fitting of artificial limbs."

I couldn't help thinking how many things went on in the world that most of us don't know exist.

We couldn't, of course, take a finished prosthesis home on the plane with us the next day. But the limb would be ready for a first fitting when we came back in three weeks for Jobi's injection of Adriamycin.

We returned to Palo Alto three weeks later with mixed emotions. Both Jobi and I were excited to see her "new leg," but Jobi was terrified of her coming injection. She sat on my lap a great deal of the time during the plane ride to California. Her tiny body seemed weightless as she nestled into my arms. She fell asleep halfway through the trip, her wig sliding down over her ear. I pulled a blanket over her, and I could feel her heart beating against her ribs.

I was unpacking a few of our clothes shortly after we arrived at the hospital when Jobi hurried into the room, her crutches tapping on the marble floor.

"Mom," she cried, tears beginning to form in her eyes, "Jo Anna is so sick. She won't talk to me."

With a sense of dread, I pushed Jobi's crooked wig straight on her head and sat her on her bed.

"Why don't you stay here a minute and play with your Barbie dolls. I'll go check it out."

She agreed tearfully, but it was Mrs. Beasly she was hugging when I left, not Barbie.

I walked into Jo Anna's room and my stomach jumped into my throat. Jo Anna Painter lay on a pillow in the red wagon kept on the floor for the children to play with. She had lost all her curly brown hair in the three weeks since we'd seen her and was painfully thin. Her eyes appeared sunken into her cheeks in the middle of dark circles. Lee, Jo Anna's plump rosy-cheeked mother, sat in a chair next to her holding her hand. Jo Anna was sobbing and moaning, a steady keening wail of misery. There was an I.V. unit next to her; the tubing that led to the needle in her arm rested midway in a large pan of water. A nurse was pouring more water into the pan, and I could tell from the steam, it was hot.

"Lee . . . what is it? What's wrong?" I asked, horrified

at Jo Anna's obvious suffering. No child should have looked so ancient. Lee's usually snapping dark eyes were sad and lifeless.

"We're warming up her medication," she said dully, not really focusing on my face. "This stuff they're trying hurts her so much when it enters the veins, they thought warming it up might help."

"How long has she been like this?" I asked, stooping to smooth Jo Anna's forehead gently. Jo Anna didn't seem to know I was there. She kept her eyes screwed tightly shut and cried steadily.

"Two days, I think," answered Lee in a disoriented manner. "She's never been so bad before." I could hear in Lee's voice the sound of defeat.

"She'll be all right, Lee. You've got to think positively. Jo Anna will get better."

"That's not what the doctors say," said Lee Painter.

I left her and returned to Jobi. I reassured her that her friend Jo Anna was having a rough time today, but was bound to be better in a few days, but the words "that's not what the doctors say" echoed in my head.

The next twenty-four hours were spent helping Jobi get through her treatment. By the time she stopped retching and gagging from Adriamycin, Jo Anna had been temporarily released from her I.V. unit, and the girls were able to play a quiet game of checkers together.

I sat watching their game, exhausted from staying up all night with Jobi. She often seemed to recover from these nights of illness more quickly than I. The head nurse, Paula, came into the room.

"There's good news and there's bad news," she quipped.

I looked up, mustering a tired smile.

"The good news is that Jobi's prosthesis is ready for fitting."

Jobi perked up. "I'm getting a new leg, Jo Anna."

"Hey, that's neat," Jo Anna replied, making a double jump over Jobi's checkers.

"Rats," Jobi scowled.

"What's the bad news?" I inquired, only half caring.

Paula grew more serious. "The prosthetist who's making the limb is a real genius . . . a young man who came here from Germany and does most of the work by hand. Dr. Wilbur recommends him for all the kids. The only trouble is that his shop is in San Jose, and our van will be tied up all day today and tomorrow.

"Is it too far to take a cab?" I didn't want to waste two more days. I had known we couldn't go home until the prosthesis was complete, but I intended to keep the delay as short as possible.

"It's more than an hour ride," said Paula apologetically. "It would cost a fortune to take a cab."

Incredibly a long-haired bearded figure appeared behind Paula in the doorway.

"Hi gang," smiled my hairy cousin Paul, looking like an angel to me. "What's happening?"

"Do you know the way to San Jose?" I sang, running over to hug him.

47

PAUL DROVE US TO SAN JOSE in the musty-smelling car he always borrowed from his friend. I made a mental note to send a gift to his friend . . . perhaps a can of spray deodorizer.

We all stared in wonder at the collection of limbs, braces, and mysterious equipment overflowing shelves and tables in

218

the small prosthetic shop. Hans Dietrich, a young man with blond hair and a heavy German accent, wasted no time on amenities. He offered us some rickety chairs and disappeared into another room. Jobi's eyes were glued to a gigantic artificial leg leaning precariously against the wall. It was probably meant for a very large man, and it wore a sock and black shoe.

"Will my leg look like that?" asked Jobi fearfully.

I put my arm around her. "Of course not," I said with more confidence than I felt.

Hans returned carrying a strange object. The top was a pink plastic cone-shaped cup perched on what looked like metal pipes. Midway between the two pipes was a pink hingelike gadget. On the bottom of the lower pipe was a wooden blob that might have been considered a foot if one wasn't too particular about shape.

"Here it is," announced Hans proudly.

I gasped involuntarily. Paul stared in disbelief, and Jobi's eyes filled with tears.

"That's not my leg, Mom. Tell him—that's not my leg."

The young German prosthetist looked at us in confusion. "Something is wrong?"

I swallowed, seeing the man's feelings were hurt. "I'm afraid we expected a prosthesis that looked like . . . well, like a real leg."

His eyes lit up with understanding, and he began to laugh. "Oh," he said, slapping his knee, "you never have seen a limb when first it is made."

Realizing we weren't sharing his amusement, he wiped his eyes and came over to Jobi.

"Do not worry, young lady. I, Hans Dietrich, will make for you the most beautiful leg you have ever seen." He stooped down in front of her. "But first, you must try on the socket. When it fits just so, and the length is right for you, I will cover with wood and plastic, you will see."

Hans had Jobi stand and remove her slacks. He then put

219

powder on her stump and pulled over it a white knit sock that was open at both ends. He next removed a little plug from near the bottom of the plastic socket and told Jobi to put her stump into the open socket. Gently, he began tugging the bottom of the sock through the hole where the plug had been. Jobi had to brace herself by holding on to me and a chair as the sock pulled her flesh into the socket. Eventually the sock was pulled free—Jobi's stump resting deep into the socket—and Hans replaced the plug.

Metal pipes and all, the sight of my daughter standing without crutches brought quick tears to my eyes. Paul and I smiled happily at each other. But Jobi was not so happy.

Suddenly she let out a yelp and began to cry. "Take it off—get it off me! It hurts!"

I moved toward her in alarm, but Hans held up a hand to stop me.

"Young lady," he said calmly but firmly. "When you first wear a suction socket, the suction draws the blood to the bottom of the stump and causes discomfort. But the pain will go away. You will see."

Jobi continued to cry and plead to have the prosthesis removed, but somehow I stifled my instinct to pull it off of her. After a while, the pain eased, and Hans began to show Jobi how to walk on the limb. She wobbled, and the kneelike joint in the middle of the two pipes buckled. Hans caught Jobi before she fell and made some adjustments with a screw driver.

"Can I take it off now?" Jobi asked in a bored tone. She obviously did not share our excitement about the prosthesis.

"In a moment," promised Hans. "First I must make a tracing." He helped Jobi walk to the wall, where a piece of white paper was taped. Placing Jobi with her heel against the paper, he traced the outline of her good leg from the front and the side. He made a tracing of her foot as well, and he finished by measuring the circumference of her leg in many places.

"I will be ready for another fitting soon," said the young German at last.

"Exactly how long will it take?" I asked. "We're anxious to return home."

"Where is your home?" Hans wanted to know.

"Minnesota."

"Ah—St. Cloud," he smiled broadly. "I have relatives there. Many lakes, yah?"

Returning to the hospital as dusk fell, I realized Hans hadn't answered my question about how long it would take to finish the prosthesis.

We didn't hear from Hans Dietrich for a week, which seemed like an eon to me, but I later learned a week was record time for the making of a prosthesis.

The hospital van took us back to San Jose. We spent the whole day in Hans's strange shop. As he worked, adjusting and refining the limb, he allowed Jobi and me to watch him, explaining his actions.

He had shaped wood into a near perfect likeness of Jobi's good leg, the ankle and calf of the prosthesis measuring identically with her own. The wood covered the metal pipes and the foot was carefully shaped. The whole structure was laminated with a type of flesh-toned plastic coating.

Jobi was unhappy with the plug visible at the base of the socket area, and I couldn't help feeling disappointed when I realized the knee mechanism could be seen easily in back of the limb. But when Jobi put her pink slacks on over the prosthesis and walked to me, I exploded into tears . . . laughing and crying at once. She grinned triumphantly, and Hans beamed at the two of us. I wished fervently that David were present to share this moment with us.

We stayed at the hospital for a few more days so Jobi could work with a physical therapist and learn to walk well on her prosthesis. It turned out to be time well spent, since we never found any therapists at home who were experienced with amputee children. However, the therapists at Stanford

221

said she walked quite well for an above-knee amputee, and while she still suffered intense pain when the limb was first pulled on, the pain lasted for shorter periods with each passing day.

Jobi couldn't wear her prosthesis for more than an hour or two at a time in the beginning. She had progressed from using crutches to leaning on a cane for security, but she was a long way from agility. She could not wear her new leg on the long trip home.

It was time to leave for the airport when I realized we had a problem. How were we to get the prosthesis home with us? I could hardly throw it over my shoulder and carry it. Jobi and I laughed uproariously thinking what people would do if they saw me walking along carrying a leg.

We finally decided to put the prosthesis in a suitcase and bring it onto the plane with us. I stuffed Jobi's clothes into my larger bag and left hers free to hold the artificial limb. By bending it at the knee, it just fit into her small suitcase.

Joan Cohen had kindly volunteered to take us to the airport—a most generous offer considering the San Francisco airport was a long ride from Palo Alto. But the offer had come as no surprise. The Cohen family had encircled us with love and kindness since we had met them. Joan and Gordon and their brood of children and pets had made our trips to Palo Alto seem almost like coming home.

Approaching the stream of people lined up to pass through the security check at the airport, I felt a stab of realization. Carry-on luggage was checked and often opened before boarding. Pushing the wheelchair, I looked down at the small suitcase resting on Jobi's lap and pictured its contents. The same thought must have occurred to Jobi. She looked from the line to the suitcase and said, "Mom—I think we've got a problem." Then we both started to laugh.

We joined the line and reached the front. The security officer smiled at Jobi and began to unzip her suitcase. I gulped, trying to decide whether to tell him what was in it. His eyes widened and his mouth flew open.

"It's an artificial limb," I said weakly. I didn't dare look down at my daughter, from whose direction came stifled giggling sounds.

"Uh—right. That's fine," said the man gruffly, trying to cover his shock. "Move right on through."

48

THE BEST THERAPIST of all for Jobi was neither doctor nor technician, but childhood itself. She wanted to ride a two-wheel bike, and like other children, got on one and promptly fell. And like other children, she climbed back on and tried it again. She fell a dozen times. Her prosthesis looked as if it had barely survived a war, it was so nicked and battered, but in the end, Band-Aids flapping from knee and elbow, Jobi rode her bike.

A trampoline was donated to Olson School.

"What do you think?" asked the gym teacher nervously over the phone.

"I think she should be wrapped in cotton batting and protected like a china doll so my hair will stop turning gray," I answered. "But let her do it."

What's a sprained wrist and dislocated shoulder to an amputee child who has the rare privilege of jumping on a trampoline? Nothing—everything healed and she was jumping again in a week.

She fell off the high bars and suffered a compression fracture of the ribs. She tripped jumping rope and broke a bone in her foot. She had a bike accident and received so many cuts and abrasions, she was wrapped in bandages like a mummy. She even managed to fall off a horse and break her nose. But she walked . . . and she climbed and she hopped and she jumped, just like other children.

But most important of all to Jobi—she danced. Before her surgery, Jobi had decided she wanted to be a dancer when she grew up. She took tap and ballet lessons from the age of three on, and when she was only seven, her Aunt Bonnie got special permission for her to dance with the Park Petites dance group at a Minnesota Viking game.

Perhaps she would never dance in the *Nutcracker* at Northrup Auditorium or do the splits at a Viking game again, but Jobi made show business become alive and well in our basement. With my father as her financial backer and official photographer, Jobi put on frequent and lavish productions in our amusement room. Jobi's friends and family were given two choices . . . be in the cast or be in the audience. Judy Sher and Jonathan generally opted for the costumes and props supplied by my father and were given supporting roles to Jobi's stardom. Before adoring crowds consisting of my father, my mother, a few bound-and-gagged friends, and me, Jobi turned on her record player and forgot she had only one leg. With flowers or funny hats perched on her blond wig, cheeks rosy with my rouge and eyes sparkling, she twirled and swayed and danced to the music. Each time I watched her ecstatic face during a "performance," I remembered Cara's words, "then see her dancing."

In May, disaster struck. There was an epidemic of chicken pox at Jobi's school. I received the notice with a sinking heart. She had just finished taking her Cytoxan pills and her white count was at its lowest point. I kept her home and away from other people, but the damage had been done the week before while she was still attending school.

Jobi came down with a raging, virulent case of chicken pox. Her temperature soared to 104 degrees, and her body was covered with ugly pox. The sores were in every orifice, including her ears and mouth. She lay on the couch in the family room so I wouldn't have to keep climbing the stairs to her bedroom. The pox sores burned and itched, and her muscles and head ached, but she scarcely had the strength to cry out. I looked at her pale thin body and bald head—both covered with sores.

I had been in constant communication with Dr. McMillan since the onset of Jobi's chicken pox. A common childhood disease like chicken pox is perilous for children on chemotherapy. When Jobi's fever spiked 105 degrees, I called Dr. McMillan immediately.

"I've seen 105 and even higher on some of these kids, but I'm coming right over," he said worriedly. "I don't want you to move her at all."

He examined her carefully, saying, "Hey kiddo . . . you look terrible."

"You should see how I feel," she joked feebly.

The doctor beckoned me into the other room.

"She's bad," he said grimly. "I won't kid you."

I felt a heaviness settle upon me. I wished David were home from work. I felt as though I needed to lean on someone so I wouldn't fall.

I wet my dry lips so I could speak. "What are you going to do?"

"I'd like to try giving her zoster immune globulin. It could help . . . but there's none available in the city—I already checked."

"What do you mean, there's none available? Can't you get some somewhere?"

"The closest supply is in New York, but they have an epidemic there too. They might not give me any."

I stared at him in disbelief. "There must be something we can do."

He put his hand on my shoulder. "I can make the serum myself from the plasma of an adult who's recently recovered from shingles . . . that's a disease similar to chicken pox."

"What good is that?" I said, near hysteria. "Where would we find such a person?"

"Don't worry about that," he said vehemently. "I'll go on television and ask for a donor if I have to."

"This is crazy," I breathed. "Like some stupid B-movie."

He didn't answer for a minute. Then he began putting on his raincoat to go out in the stormy spring afternoon.

"Here's what we'll do," he said at last. "We'll wait another six hours. I'm hoping she's passing a crisis with this thing, but if her fever doesn't drop and she doesn't show any sign of improvement, I'll get that globulin . . . any way I have to."

I couldn't reach David; he was out of the office. I just sat next to Jobi most of the afternoon. I couldn't sponge her for fear of spreading the pox further on her body, though where the disease would find an inch of open space I couldn't guess. All I could do was dab tepid water on her face with cotton balls, discarding each after touching her.

As the hours passed with no change in her condition, I began to grow angry. No, I thought fiercely. I won't give her up to a goddamned childhood disease if I wouldn't give her up to cancer. I willed her to recover with all my might.

Early that evening Jobi sat up a little on the couch.

"Can I have a Popsicle?"

I looked at her in surprise. I had had to force a few drops of water into her mouth during the last two days . . . she had wanted neither food nor liquid. David, recently home from work, sat on the couch next to her.

"Let's see what your temperature is first," he said and plopped a thermometer into her mouth.

I waited anxiously. David read the thermometer and smiled.

"100.3," he said simply.

Overjoyed, I ran to the couch and hugged them both, then I hurried to call Dr. McMillan.

"Call off the TV cameras," I said happily. "Her fever broke and she's asking for Popsicles."

"What flavor?" Dr. McMillan asked seriously. "Tell her I like root beer best."

49

THE MOODY BLUES WERE NOT unknown among the children.

Most of the time, a stranger visiting the oncology wing of Children's Hospital at Stanford would be pleasantly shocked at the cheerful attitude of the young patients. The same sound of laughter and play could be heard in these halls as in any area where children are found. Granted, the laughter was often blunted by a cry or shout of protest, but the prevailing atmosphere was surprisingly lighthearted. Except occasionally, when shadows fell over small pale faces.

It was impossible to pin down the moment the aura changed or even the reason for the mood swings. One day the halls resounded with evenly distributed giggles and whines; the next day the air seemed quieter—subdued in tone. The children became visibly apathetic, their dull moods punctuated only by occasional bursts of peckishness. At such times, two children might sit quietly side by side for an hour, listlessly moving puzzle pieces. Suddenly a fight would break out. The children would shout and call each other names, sometimes even striking each other in undefined anger.

We were in Palo Alto for Jobi's injection of high-dose methotrexate on one such day; a day when the air crackled with static, and the children bristled as they passed each other in the corridor. Dr. Wilbur had an idea.

227

The hospital complex contained a therapeutic swimming pool used for the orthopedic patients in another section of the building. Dr. Wilbur decided his children would benefit from some exercise . . . exercise such as swimming.

The idea was greeted with enthusiasm by children and parents. Every child who could possibly be disconnected from I.V. units was assembled in front of the nursing station. Paula beamed at all the excited faces.

A few in the group had bathing suits. Most wore shorts and T-shirts or whatever they had with them that they didn't mind getting wet. But no one really cared what he or she wore so long as they were among the privileged gang who were going swimming.

What a strange sight we must have made as we walked through the halls of the Children's Hospital at Stanford. The head nurse, Paula, led, her limp pronounced, her brown hair bouncing jauntily as she stepped down on her polio-twisted leg. Paula held the pudgy hand of Sarah, whose nearly bald head still displayed the marking pen artwork of nuclear medicine. The brace on the girl's leg made the rhythm of her gait different from Paula's, and the two walked in counterpoint harmony.

Behind them came the unholy three. Tall, handsome Michael, swinging powerfully on his crutches, seemed unconscious of his amputation, now showing below his gym shorts. Robbie Denton had mysteriously retained his fine blond hair despite massive doses of leukemia-fighting drugs, and a shock of it hung over his pale forehead. Robbie pushed his friend Carl in a wheelchair, demonstrating an occasional wheely as he lifted the front wheels off the ground. Overweight Carl preferred the chair to crutches. He had been fitted for an artificial limb, but he refused to wear it, claiming it "ain't worth the bother." Carl had lost all his hair, and he was now a bizarre caricature of the roughly good-looking teenager I had met my first day at the hospital.

Jobi and Laurel Sardi followed the boys, who studiously ignored them. Jobi was wearing her short curly wig today, and had caught back a lock of it with a purple barrette. She wore a lavender smock over her shorts, one bare tennis-shoed leg striding on one side, on the other, only space. Laurel's dark hair swung from its ponytail as she pranced to keep up with Jobi, who moved more quickly on crutches than her younger friend could walk. Laurel was back in the hospital only for a checkup and would leave the next day.

Four mothers, Emily, Lois, Maureen, and I, followed the children, carrying towels and robes. Emily and Lois never took their eyes from their sons, Robbie and Michael. It was almost as if by watching them vigilantly they hoped to prevent anything bad from happening to the two boys. I understood their feelings. There were times I caught myself watching Jobi breathe at night.

Maureen Sardi walked next to me. She was relaxed now that Laurel was out of danger and no longer needing even the sling on her arm. Behind us trailed Natasha, the Russian immigrant, foreign-looking with her hair in a bun and wearing a paisley shawl. Still nervous and high strung, she clutched the arm of her son, Ivan. Natasha nearly smothered twelve-year-old Ivan with protection. Ivan, like so many of the others, had no hair; he wore a shiny black wig that was much too large for him. His Hodgkin's disease was responding to treatment, but no one knew for how long.

Behind us staggered a weary Irene, pushing little Chris in a stroller. This was Irene's day off from her double-waitress job, and usually she spent it sleeping. But Chris was being the most ornery of all the children lately, whining and howling as only an unhappy three-year-old can, and Irene was hoping a swim would sweeten his temper. Irene swore softly as she tripped over the hem of the Oriental kimono she wore, and Chris alternately sucked his thumb and emitted staccato screeches that echoed down the corridor.

Will Painter walked slowly at the end of our parade. Jo Anna had retreated far into herself of late, and she rarely spoke. Will held his daughter's reluctant hand firmly and pulled her along, talking to her cheerfully even though she didn't answer him. Jo Anna was very ill, and her swollen white face and round belly reflected the strong doses of medication being used to try and save her.

Strangers watching might have shuddered at the sight of our group, but if they closed their eyes and listened, they would have heard the sounds of any gathering of people heading for the ole swimming hole.

"Robbie—now you quit bouncin' Carl around like that, y'all hear?" called Emily. "You're gonna throw him clean outta that chair."

"He likes it, Ma," Robbie hollered. "Don't ya, Carl?"

"Cut it out, will ya, Denton?" demanded Carl.

"Come on, you weasels," teased Michael. "I'll race you to the water."

"Watch out, you guys. Don't knock anyone over." Paula laughed as the boys raced past her.

"Far out," commented Sarah excitedly.

"Wait for me, Jobi," pleaded Laurel. "I can't go so fast."

"I can't wait to swim." Jobi beamed. "I swam in Hawaii in the ocean."

"In the ocean?" breathed Laurel with admiration. "My mother only lets me go in the wading pool in our backyard."

"That's cause you're just a little kid," explained the nine-year-old wisely. "She'll let you go in the ocean when you're older."

"Who've we got for bridge tonight?" asked Lois, lighting a cigarette as we walked, even though smoking in the halls was forbidden.

"Are you staying overnight, Maureen?" I asked hopefully.

"Sure am. Nick won't be back for us until tomorrow morning after Laurel's X rays."

"Then we're set." I smiled.

"Ah'll bring the cards. I got me a new deck," offered

230

Emily, smiling too. Without a bridge game, evenings could not be borne. Even Lois, who rarely smiled, looked pleased.

"Ivan, you must not stay in the water long. You will catch a chill," instructed Natasha, her accent thick.

"All right, Mother," Ivan agreed politely. He never fought his mother's ministrations, seeming to sense she needed to take care of him for her own survival.

"Don't pick your nose, Chris, it ain't polite." Irene's hoop earrings shook with the impact of her jaws vigorously chewing a wad of gum. "Shit," she added as she tripped on her kimono again.

"Now honey, you're just going to have a wonderful time swimming," boomed Will Painter. "You'll splash and play with the kids and feel real good—you'll see."

Jo Anna didn't answer.

The smell of chlorine greeted us before we actually saw the swimming pool. Steps quickened. The pool was in a large room with one windowed wall; the other three were cement blocks. The pool itself was not big, perhaps ten feet by twenty feet, but the children approached it as eagerly as though it were of olympic proportions.

Crutches and wheelchairs were abandoned, and everyone got into the water as best and as fast as he or she could.

I slid into the water gingerly, waiting for the little shock of cold even heated pools provide. Luxurious warmth surrounded me instead. I had known this was a therapeutic pool, but hadn't realized the water would be nearly hot.

"Jobi—this is like a bathtub. Come on in," I called.

She laughed with delight and sat on the edge of the pool. I held my arms up to her and she jumped. I hugged her bony little body to me with one quick squeeze and lowered her into the water. She had warned me in advance that she wouldn't take off her wig.

"I won't go in if I can't keep my wig on, Mom," she had said stubbornly as we were deciding which of our clothing could withstand a dunk in chlorinated water.

I looked at her in surprise. At home she came in the door from school and tossed the wig on the nearest chair. Of course, only a select few friends like Dana and Judy and Julie were allowed to see her without the wig, but I didn't expect her to be self-conscious at the hospital.

"But Sunshine," I protested, "half the kids here have lost their hair."

"I don't care. I want to keep my wig on—please, Mom." Tears were pooling in her eyes.

I sighed. "Okay, love. If the thing turns green, we'll save it for St. Patrick's Day."

Now I helped her balance as she splashed in the water, all grin and wet wig. Around us the children laughed and played, screeching loudly to hear their voices echo off the water and walls. Will Painter and I were the only parents in the pool, but Paula scrambled after a ball with the boys. It was amazing how powerfully Michael could swim. I thought it was because his arms were strong from using his crutches. Carl just squatted in the shallow end, letting the waves made by the rowdier swimmers splash over him. He resembled a smiling, waterlogged Buddha.

I held Jobi under her stomach, and she pretended to swim. Sarah, who would not leave the side of the pool, called a friendly, "Far out," and hit the water with the flat of her hand, causing a clapping sound that seemed to delight her.

Laurel kept calling on her mother to watch her. Securing Maureen's attention, the little girl screwed her eyes shut tightly and pinched her nose with two plump fingers.

"One, two, three," she counted loudly and dunked herself under the water. She jumped up again before the water even closed over her head and waited for Maureen's applause.

Will coaxed his daughter to unwrap her arms from around his neck. Jo Anna clung to her father, her head on his shoulder. Will smiled and spoke to her as though she were having a good time.

"Hey now, here we go," he chortled, dunking them both

into the water. Finally he persuaded Jo Anna to climb on his back, and he paddled around the pool, laughing in spite of Jo Anna's silence.

Irene could not even persuade her reluctant son to go into the water. As she walked toward the edge of the pool with Chris in her arms, he had begun to cry and struggle to get away from her. She gave up with a grimace of disgust and plunked him back in his stroller.

"I could have been sleeping, you little monster," she informed him. Chris put his thumb in his mouth and regarded her solemnly. She bent and kissed him, leaving a smear of purplish lipstick on his cheek.

After a half hour had passed, I noticed the noise level in the pool had decreased considerably. The shouting echo games had ceased, and no one was splashing anybody else. I felt a little sluggish and decided to get out of the water. I left Jobi holding hands with Laurel and dried myself off, keeping an eye on the pool. I saw Paula throw up her hands in defeat and leave the water too.

Soon Will swam over to where I was sitting at the edge of the pool and set Jo Anna next to me.

"Whew," exclaimed the huge man, clambering out of the water with obvious difficulty. "I feel rung out."

"I know. I'm pooped too," I agreed. "It must be old age."

Ivan had been swimming laps back and forth across the length of the pool. Natasha followed him, walking along the decking, never taking her anxious eyes from her son. Now I saw her lean against the side wall and remove her shawl. Ivan turned over on his back and floated, his eyes closed.

Emily, Maureen, and Lois came to sit by the pool with Will and me.

"It is hotter in here than South Car'lina in the summer time," protested Emily.

"Tell me about it," said Lois, perspiration beading her upper lip.

"How long do you think they ought to swim?" wondered Maureen.

I looked up at the clock on the wall. "They've only been in the water about forty-five minutes."

"They sure aren't going to get chilled," Will quipped and we all laughed.

Within another ten minutes, the quiet in the pool grew more pronounced. Activity also lessened, and soon I realized the children were, for the most part, merely standing in the water and trailing their hands aimlessly.

I rose and went over to the other end of the pool where Paula was drying her hair with a towel.

"These kids are awfully quiet," I said.

"I was just thinking that. I guess they've had enough." Paula stood awkwardly and limped to the pool. "Okay, guys —everybody out."

The swimmers gave a few token groans of disappointment, but made their way to the edges without further protest. Carl didn't move. He appeared to have fallen asleep sitting in the water and was snoring loudly. The rest of the children moved slowly and seemed to be without strength. Michael pulled himself out of the water and sat limply on the side. The others just stood in the water at the edge, their faces slack.

"What's wrong with them?" I asked Paula. She frowned and watched Robbie being pulled out of the water by a straining Emily.

"The water," Paula said finally. "The hot water. I should have known."

"What do you mean?" asked Maureen, who had come near to hear what we were discussing.

"This pool is therapeutic—it's for kids with bone and muscle problems. The water temperature is about a hundred degrees. Patients are put in the water for ten or fifteen minutes at a time . . . to relax their muscles."

I started to laugh. "Well, they sure are relaxed."

Everyone looked where I pointed. Sarah was now stretched out on the pool decking, flat on her back with her arms and legs splayed.

"Ten or fifteen minutes . . ." breathed Maureen, suddenly realizing what Paula meant. "Our kids have been in the water close to an hour."

Paula nodded and laughed with me. "I think we may have discovered the answer to tranquilizers. Come on—we better get the rest of them from the pool before they all pass out."

Fishing the children from the water was like dredging for rubber tires. By now the remaining swimmers were limp and didn't even help us pull them out. It took Michael, Emily, Lois, and me to drag Carl onto the decking.

"Man, I need a nap," he said quickly and curled up by the pool.

"Not here, you don't," warned Paula, bringing his wheelchair over and demanding he get in it.

Our bedraggled troupe undoubtedly resembled losers of a war as we slogged through the halls back to our own ward. Even the parents who hadn't been in the water were damp, disheveled, and exhausted.

As I pulled off Jobi's soggy wig, I was pleased to note it was still blond, if a little stringy. I had to lift her up and put her into bed, she was so tired. But she smiled serenely as her eyes closed.

"Can we go swimming again tomorrow?"

I had a feeling Dr. Wilbur's plan to calm down the children would be scrapped and labeled "Overkill." But the moody blues seemed to disappear for a long time after that.

50

THE MORNING AFTER OUR SWIM, I met the Gonzalez family and became aware of the gross financial difficulties besetting many of the children's parents. Because Jobi was on a protocol study, the costs of her hospital stay, doctors' fees, and medications were paid by the state of California. A special travel fund even provided half of our costly air fares.

The major portion of children at the hospital were not so lucky. The very poor patients qualified for government aid; their expenses were drastically reduced. The very rich needed to make sacrifices in their life-styles, but were able to survive the astronomical expenses acquired through prolonged illness. But the middle-income families, their incomes not low enough to qualify for aid nor high enough to pay the bills, were devastated.

Marie and Frank Gonzales came under the latter category. Immigrants from Mexico, the young couple came to the United States to make a better life for themselves. Marie worked long hours so Frank could attend school and receive his degree in engineering. After graduation, Frank secured a good job, and Marie began producing their long awaited family. Three little Gonzalezes followed in three successive years. Life was good for the Gonzalez family and the future promised the fulfillment of all their dreams.

And then five-year-old Tony Gonzalez contracted leukemia. The disease lingered, the expenses mounted. Frank watched his salary disappear before his eyes. Still the bills poured in. There was not enough money to pay them and

236

feed and clothe his wife and other two children. In despair, Frank Gonzalez quit his job, destroying the career he and Marie had invested years to attain. Carrying out his desperate plan, he declared bankruptcy and applied for government aid to pay his son's medical expenses. Finally poor enough, he received it.

The story made me furious. Something was wrong with a society that allowed such a thing to happen. But the world was full of strange injustice. Jobi was a victim of similarly perverse logic.

To the best of our knowledge, the twin cities of Minneapolis and St. Paul had only one source of aid for an amputee child in 1973. Shriners Hospital for Crippled Children in St. Paul was the one facility we could find where physical therapists had experience with amputee children. We had applied for the out-patient therapy program as soon as we returned home from California with Jobi's new prosthesis.

The answer shocked and appalled me. Shriners Hospital rejected Jobi as a therapy patient. They based their decision on two facts: they refused to accept a child with catastrophic disease into their already crowded program, and David made too much money to qualify for their free-patient-care plan, the only plan they had.

"Are you telling me they won't help her because she has cancer?" I asked David, my voice almost a screech.

He nodded miserably. His father was very active in the Shrine, but even he could not get the Shriners Hospital authorities to change their minds.

"Tell them we'll pay," I had begged David. "We don't need free care."

"I tried that," he said angrily. "They won't take you if you can pay."

I raged and raved at the terrible injustice that prevented my child from getting the care she needed. But to no avail. Ultimately, the only valuable therapy Jobi ever received was

237

from the prosthetists at the Winkly Company where Jobi's artificial limbs were subsequently made and serviced in Minneapolis.

During our many stays at Children's Hospital at Stanford, I had watched several of the mothers give their children injections. Before Jobi's I.V. of methotrexate was even started in May, I sought out Dr. Wilbur.

"I want to give Jobi the rescue injections myself," I told him. "That way I can take her home immediately after she's through with her methotrexate."

I was still obsessed with the idea that Jobi didn't get as sick when she was at home. If I planned things right, she could recover from methotrexate surrounded by her friends and family. Also, I wanted to spend more time at home for Heidi's sake.

I hadn't realized just how deeply Heidi's resentment of Jobi had manifested itself until one morning between trips to Palo Alto. I was polishing my nails when Heidi came stomping into my room. Her cheeks were flushed, and her blue eyes crackled fire behind her glasses.

"You have to do something about Jo Beth." Heidi spat out her sister's name as though it tasted bad.

"What's wrong, honey?" I asked.

"Everything—all her!" Heidi's nostrils flared in anger.

"What's bothering you?" I asked again, trying to be patient.

"Tell her to keep her robe buttoned up," Heidi demanded, nearly in tears.

"Her robe? Heidi, I want to help you, but I don't know what you're talking about."

"She leaves her robe open and I can see her skin."

I stared at my daughter, speechless.

"Her skin is so white," Heidi nearly shrieked. "It makes me sick. She's ugly!"

238

Before I could respond, Heidi whirled and ran out of my room. I heard a door slam and muffled crying.

I didn't know what to do. Surely it was normal for sisters to have fights, but Heidi and Jobi had so much more ammunition than most sisters.

The afternoon before, all three children had been playing in the backyard. Jobi and Jon were in the sandbox, and Heidi decided to join them. The weather was mild, but the sand was still wet and heavy from a recently departed winter.

I was digging in a flower garden in front of the house, so I could just hear the children if I listened, or tune them out, which is what I chose to do for a few minutes.

Suddenly the noise level rose and childish voices broke through my fragile sound barrier.

"Quit throwing sand or I'll tell." Jobi's voice.

"You started it, you big baby." Heidi.

"I did not, fatso!"

"Who are you calling fat . . . baldy!"

A shriek had hurtled itself through the air followed by shouting and crying.

Jonathan came running around the side of the house, his face and shirt liberally decorated with wet sand.

"You better come, Mommy. I think they're killing each other," the little boy had said happily.

I was already on my feet, and as I headed for the backyard, Jobi's screeching changed pitch and transcended even her sister's powerful barrage.

"Ow—ow—it's them . . . they're back; the phantom pains."

I lifted her out of the sandbox. She had flung her prosthesis into the grass to play more comfortably, so the lifting was easy.

"It's like a car is running over my foot, Mom," she had cried, burying her sandy face in my hair.

"Liar!" shouted Heidi. The clumps of wet sand clinging to her hands bore witness to her involvement in the sand fight. "She didn't have phantom pains before. She just wants to get me in trouble again. Jobi, you're nothing but a faker!"

"Heidi, please stop shouting. Jobi, you must calm down. I'll take you inside and give you some aspirin." I started toward the house.

"Sure—take care of her. Don't worry about me," Heidi pouted.

"Are you hurt?" I had asked her.

She had turned her face away from me.

The sand fight of the day before still in my mind, I followed Heidi to her room after she fled from mine. I knocked on the door.

"Go away," she wailed.

I went in anyway. I sat on the edge of her double bed and reached out to stroke the hair streaming across her face. She rolled away from my touch and sat up.

"Talk to me," I begged.

"I have nothing to say." Her face was set stubbornly, and she wiped tears with the back of her hand.

"Why are you so angry with Jobi?" No answer. "We have to go back to California in two days—I don't like leaving you like this."

"I think you do like leaving. I think you both like it a lot." Heidi challenged.

"What makes you think there's anything to like about it? Heidi, it's a hospital—everyone's sick there, and sometimes they die. It's horrible."

"Oh yeah? And how about the Cohens and all their neat animals . . . is that horrible?"

"Heidi . . ." I tried to explain.

"And Paul and Cindy. I know you stay in California longer than you have to just so you can have fun with Paul and Cindy."

"Honey, that's not true. Believe me."

But she hadn't believed me. The next morning, lying on

240

the kitchen table was a piece of paper with Heidi's childish writing on it; a sort of poem.

The poem said:

> Jobi has no heart.
> Jobi has no soul.
> Jobi has no leg.

I threw it away.

I was appalled and frustrated at the same time. Obviously, Heidi's need for my attention was growing, yet there was no lessening of Jobi's dependence on me. I knew I would have to find time for both, but I didn't know if I could find the strength.

Heidi's poem echoed in my mind as I sat facing Dr. Wilbur in his office. My face must have reflected the urgency of my need to return home quickly, because Dr. Wilbur offered little resistance to my request to learn how to give Jobi her rescue injections.

"You know Jobi has to be injected every three hours for twenty-four hours," Dr. Wilbur reminded me. "You'll have to be up all night."

"I know. I can do it."

"All right," he agreed. "I'll have Paula show you how it's done."

It wasn't as simple as it looked. The rescue had to be mixed and drawn into the syringe, which had to be tapped and carefully checked for air bubbles. No air must be allowed into the vein. Another syringe had to be prepared with heparin. Heparin was injected after the rescue to keep the vein open. The whole process may have been routine to a nurse, but to me it was monumental. I never gave Jobi the injection without breaking into a cold sweat. She, of course, didn't care who put the needle into the tube leading to her arm—as long as she could push the plunger.

I harassed the poor staff at Stanford to do everything according to my tight time schedule. I had planned all the injections so I would have to give Jobi only one rescue during the trip home.

I practically pulled the I.V. out of her arm myself when I saw the last drop of methotrexate enter the tubing. Paula laughed at my anxiety.

"Relax. You're a pro now. Everything will be fine."

A hospital volunteer drove us to the airport. I kept looking at my watch, worried I would miss the first injection. Jobi was not yet nauseated from the methotrexate, but I knew it would happen before long. The trick was to get her home first.

As the plane took off, Jobi was becoming listless, a sure sign the nausea would not be long in coming. For once I didn't coax her to eat or drink. Until we were safely home, the less there was in her stomach, the better.

I pulled the carefully wrapped syringe from my purse. It was time to administer the rescue. Paula had prepared the syringes for me and filled them with the two solutions for easy use on the plane. Once home I would have to fill them myself.

A new fear thrust itself into my mind. What if the needle that had been placed in Jobi's vein at the hospital came out? What would I do? Her arm looked all right, but it could come out as I injected the rescue into the tube leading to the needle in her vein.

My hands shook a little as I poised the needle. Jobi looked at me trustingly. Her utter faith in me and total acceptance of my decisions from the very beginning had both warmed and frightened me. I knew most young children have blind faith in their parents, but rarely was that faith tested on such life-and-death matters.

I inserted the needle and Jobi pushed the plunger. Everything was as it should be. Sighing with relief, I put the equipment away and took Jobi on my lap. She cuddled in

242

my arms and we put our heads together and softly sang a little song from a show I had written for children called "The Misfit Wizard." The wizard sang:

> Here I am; I'm a flop among wizards.
> I try evil potions to make.
> I add bat wings and gizzards of lizards;
> All I get is a nice chocolate cake.

I added the evil potion—I was hoping for the chocolate cake.

51

OUR TRIPS TO PALO ALTO were getting Jobi and me down. Jobi was lonely at the hospital. Her friend, Jo Anna Painter, was too sick to play with Jobi most of the time, and my nine-year-old daughter seemed instinctively to shy away from making new attachments. Only Rachel Cohen could entice her to be her happy self when we were in Palo Alto. But most of the time Jobi had to be in the hospital where Rachel wasn't allowed to visit, so the sunshiny smiles I was used to seeing were rare.

I found the hospital oppressive. There were frequent deaths, and the silence when a room suddenly emptied was terrifying. I tried to make no new friends, and I didn't ask about my old ones if they weren't there. The answers were often too painful.

In June we were in Palo Alto for Jobi's injection of Adriamycin. On the bulletin board near the nursing station, I saw a notice of a meeting for parents whose children had cancer. I considered going, but suddenly a door slammed shut and my mind said no. I could no longer be the company for everyone's misery. I believed Jobi was getting well, and I decided not to identify with a group of parents with sick children.

"Is there any reason Jobi can't have her methotrexate at home when it's time?" I asked Dr. Wilbur, whom I had cornered in a hallway.

"You mean in a hospital in Minneapolis?" he asked, a small twinkle in his eye. "I'm beginning to think you don't like it here."

"You're right," I laughed. "I don't. Dr. Wilbur, can't Dr. McMillan or someone give Jobi the drug? Methotrexate isn't being used exclusively on the protocol study, so it must be obtainable at Minneapolis."

Dr. Wilbur looked thoughtful and smiled. "I don't see why it can't be arranged. Of course you realize you'll have to incur the expenses yourself for any treatment not done in this hospital."

I nodded. I was sure David would agree. No doubt our insurance would cover some of the expense and the cost of our half of the air fare should make up the difference.

A nurse at St. Anthony Hospital wrote about me on Jobi's chart: "Overly anxious mother." Perhaps she was right, but she didn't know about the unspoken pact I had made with my daughter. She endured every ordeal I told her was necessary, and I never made her face any of them alone.

Jobi had completed her Cytoxan pills at home and gotten another clear chest X ray. Now it was the first of August and time for her methotrexate treatment. As promised, Dr. Wilbur arranged for it to be done at St. Anthony Hospital in Minneapolis. St. Anthony—where it had all begun. Could it have been only a little over eight months ago? It seemed like most of my life.

The staff on pediatrics at St. Anthony remembered Jobi

Halper. But they hadn't expected to see her alive again. Nurses and aides and even custodial people came to say hello to her. She was put in a small intensive care room—not, at her request, the same room where she'd recovered from surgery.

The next morning, a young female staff doctor came to place the I.V. needle in a vein. I lost an argument over whether the needle would be of a type to accommodate heparin. I didn't want Jobi tied to the I.V. unit, even though all the rescues would be administered in the hospital this time. But the doctor refused to use the heparin lock method, insisting that type of needle came out of the vein too easily. Knowing the heparin lock was used successfully in Palo Alto all the time, I began to protest, but I realized Jobi was becoming agitated during the discussion. Anticipation of the needle was hard enough on her; no useful purpose was being served by delaying the injection for a debate.

During the middle of the night, the needle that the young doctor had insisted was safer infiltrated Jobi's vein and had to be removed. I had left firm instructions that I was to be called in case there were any problems. Jobi refused to allow a new needle to be placed in her arm unless I was with her. David drove me to St. Anthony Hospital at three o'clock in the morning. I cried with Jobi as another doctor tried to find a good vein.

Throughout the past eight and a half months, Jobi had remained cheerful and compliant. I gave her many conversational openings to complain or protest her lot. But other than crying out from the pain of the needles, she held back any sign of self-pity.

The next day her dam broke. The needle fell out again with only two rescue injections left to administer. Another vein would have to be found for the I.V. needle. Hearing the news, Jobi began to cry. Her sobs sounded more like those of a woman than a child. I couldn't seem to comfort her.

Dr. Parrish came into the room. I hadn't seen Josephine Parrish for a while, and her shining, open face was a welcome sight.

"What's going on?" she asked over Jobi's sobs.

"The needle came out of her vein for the second time," I explained. "She's very upset."

Dr. Parrish sat on the bed next to Jobi and gathered her onto her lap. Jobi buried her face in the woman's shoulder and whimpered, "Why is this all happening to me, Dr. Parrish? I must be the unluckiest little girl in the whole world."

I felt I was coming apart when I heard her words. Dr. Parrish saw my face and told me I should go for a walk. She wanted to speak to Jobi alone.

One of my good friends, Patti Abrams, was in the hall waiting to see me. Her vivacious chatter was just what I needed to fight the terrible depression threatening to overwhelm me.

I don't know what Dr. Parrish said to Jobi as she held her in her arms that day, but when I returned, my daughter was smiling again and the tears didn't come back again for a long time.

I had one more plan requiring Dr. Wilbur's support. I wanted Jobi to receive Adriamycin in Minneapolis and eliminate further trips to California. When Jobi was at home, she took a day or two to recover from a drug and then returned to school or play as though nothing had happened. In Palo Alto, she became one of the sick children there, and her low spirits lingered for days.

Dr. Wilbur was not so easy to convince. Adriamycin was the key to the whole protocol study, and it could not be used anywhere else in the country until California's study was complete.

I was seated in Wilbur's office staring at the cat on the poster. Déja vù, I thought. I wasn't sure I ever wanted to see a picture of a cat again when this was all over.

246

Jobi and I had just arrived in Palo Alto for her Adriamycin treatment. We had stopped for a day in Salt Lake City to visit our old friends, the Sardis, on the way to Palo Alto. Laurel was healed and thriving and we had a pleasant stay, including a dip in the Great Salt Lake. Somehow the stopover in Salt Lake City made our arrival at the hospital, the world of needles and sickness, bleaker than ever.

"I'll be honest with you, Mrs. Halper," said Dr. Wilbur with a frown. "I don't see how I can send Adriamycin out of here. If I were a doctor in Minneapolis and I had a patient dying of cancer, and there sitting on the shelf was a potentially life-saving drug, I'd use it and protocol study be damned. Then what happens to our carefully planned and documented study . . . and what happens to Jobi?"

"I see what you mean," I sighed. "But there must be a way."

"Let me think about it," he said. "I'll get back to you."

An hour before we were to leave for home, Dr. Wilbur sent for me. I entered his office eagerly . . . I just knew he wouldn't let me down.

"Here's the plan," he said without preface. "About a week before Jobi's next Adriamycin treatment is due, I'll have it sent by special delivery to the Minneapolis airport. You or your husband will have to pick it up there and sign for it. Then you must take it home with you, and not let it out of your sight until the people at St. Anthony are ready to mix and inject it."

"Wow," I chuckled. "I feel like I'm working for the C.I.A."

"I know," he laughed with me. "But I have people I must answer to, and this is the only plan that makes them comfortable. I might add, they weren't too thrilled with a patient on the study receiving all the treatments in another state."

"We'll do exactly as you say," I broke in quickly. "I personally guarantee the Adriamycin will be used only for Jobi."

My heart sang as we completed discussing the arrangements. I would have to bring Jobi to Palo Alto one more time for complete X rays and tests at the end of her year of chemotherapy. But that wouldn't be until January, and this was still summer. These days my thoughts were focused on November, when Jobi would have survived for one year, and on the promise of renewed hope in her recovery.

52

NOVEMBER . . . a year had passed since the evening Jobi held out a slim, tanned leg and said, "A boy kicked me."

It was afternoon—the gray, leafless, bleak kind of an afternoon only a Minnesota November can produce. There was no snow yet, but the air was damp and cold. Jobi wasn't home from school yet.

I stayed home most of the time. I was afraid to leave for fear the school would try to reach me or the snow would come and Jobi would be stranded. She insisted on walking to and from school instead of riding. I allowed it so long as she had friends with her. I knew Dana would walk home with her, but even Dana couldn't help Jobi walk on ice and snow.

Jobi was becoming more and more agile with her new prosthesis. The first one had been long since outgrown. Jobi's rapid growth was causing great problems for her body and for the prosthetists at the Winkley Company, where her artificial limbs were made and serviced.

Typical of the amputee child, her back began to show signs of scoliosis, a curvature of the spine. It was during the growth years the condition usually worsened, so she must be x-rayed and watched carefully. If the curvature became too great, it could mean a body brace or even surgery.

Al Pike, the prosthetist at the Winkley Company, was ready to tear his hair out over her growth pattern.

"I no more than add an inch to the bottom when she's outgrown the socket," he moaned.

The cost of a prosthesis at that time was between eight and nine hundred dollars. David's insurance covered the cost of one prosthesis per year, but Jobi needed two or even three in that amount of time, plus other adjustments and work. David moaned right along with Al Pike everytime she grew an inch or put on a pound.

Jobi and I spent a great deal of time at the Winkley Company, as they not only worked on her limb, but taught her how to walk.

"Now take that little hop out of your walk—don't be in such a hurry," Al Pike would tell her. "Quit bouncing."

Jobi would laugh and put a book on her head to show Al how smoothly she could walk if she wished. Her admiring companions, Dana or Judy or Julie Schwantes, would laugh with her and applaud.

Julie was a year younger than Jobi and Judy, but such a warm, friendly little girl, they couldn't help liking her and making her their friend. Julie often sat with Jobi's head in her lap when she was sick from chemotherapy.

"I like playing house with you, Jobi," Julie would say, stroking the pale fuzz on Jobi's head. "You look just like a real baby."

I watched the wind blow some dead leaves up the street. The house was very still at two in the afternoon with the children at school. I tried to concentrate on the outline I was making for a new show, but I stared at the words, "Act I, Scene 1," and nothing else came into my mind. It had been over twenty-four hours since Jobi's chest X ray had been taken, and I still didn't know the results. You'd think after a year of these torturous waits for X-ray results, I'd be used to them. But I wasn't . . . especially not today, November 15.

Exactly one year before, Dr. Eugene Pelletier had looked

at me impassively and told me there would be a tumor in Jobi's lung within one year. And then she would die. The doctor's prognosis had been brief and to the point. There was no room for comfort; there was no space for hope.

Why didn't the medical center call? Perhaps the X rays showed the tumor had appeared in Jobi's lung, and they were waiting for Dr. McMillan to be free to call and break the news. Perhaps . . .

The phone rang and I jumped.

"Mrs. Halper? This is Jane from Dr. McMillan's office. Jobi's X rays look fine."

I thanked her and replaced the receiver on the phone. Sudden tears welled in my eyes. "Well, now what are you crying about?" I asked myself. "Because I almost listened to him," I answered.

I meant Dr. Pelletier and all the other doctors like him who were so generous with the bitter truth and so stingy with a touch of hope. What good does it do anyone in this world to give up? What battle can be won without a fight? What race can be finished if you quit before you begin?

I put my head down on my arms and cried out loud as I saw Dr. Pelletier's face; heard him saying, "Osteogenic sarcoma reappears in the lung . . . there is no treatment . . . her chances are slim. . . ." Then I saw Dr. Jordan Wilbur and listened to him say, "We never give up . . . we form a circle of hope, love, and protection around each child."

I closed my eyes. "Thank God," I whispered, "I opted for the hope and had the strength to pursue it."

EPILOGUE

FOUR YEARS AFTER I had watched the windy November day and waited for the results of Jobi's twelfth X ray, a celebration was held.

We knew Jobi's chances of surviving osteogenic sarcoma had increased dramatically after one disease-free year, but the doctors had told us that no cancer patient is considered cured until five years after the onset of illness. On November 15, 1976, our family gathered to celebrate the day we could call her cured.

I set the dining room table with my best china. I was glad the party would take place in the dining room, with its soft yellow carpeting and walls and its tinkling crystal chandelier. The room reminded me of Jobi somehow; delicate, fragile, but filled with warmth, light and a quiet strength.

Carefully, I laid a snowy linen napkin at the place where each member of my family would sit that night. Bauby would sit at one end of the table. Still strong and bright at seventy-six, she was sure her prayers to Zady had saved Jobi's life. Who could say she was wrong?

Next to her would sit my mother. She hadn't changed in appearance over the years. Her hair was thick and lovely, her skin smooth and fine. But inside, she would never be the same. No more the flighty social butterfly, her experiences had made her a woman of depth. I respected my mother more than I had ever thought possible, and we had become friends. When she took my father's hand during dinner tonight, which I was sure she would do, it would not be to lean on him, but to share her joy with him.

Jonathan would sit next to his grandfather. Jon was not a baby any longer. The tall, dark nine-year-old was already strongly muscled and had made more than one touchdown on the football field that fall. If he had been affected by the events of the past five years, it seemed only in that he was not as young as most nine-year-olds. He had had to examine the value of life very early in his own.

I recalled one day when Jonathan and his friend, Mike Midlo, were sitting on the front steps talking. I could hear them through the open door. Mike's younger sister had died several months before, and his mother had told me he wouldn't talk about it.

"I think I'll be a baseball player when I grow up," said Jon, bouncing his ball in a glove.

"Yeah, me too," decided Mike promptly.

"Course, I don't know. I like acting in plays too. My mom let me be in one of her shows."

"I like shows a lot. It's like all that modeling I did last year. It was fun."

"My mom says I should be a writer 'cause I write good stories," considered Jonathan.

"Yeah? No kiddin'. I like to write stories too," exclaimed Mike.

"We sure are a lot alike," decided Jonathan.

"Yeah."

There was a pause as two young minds drifted in other directions.

"We even both have sisters who had cancer," Jon said finally.

"Uh-huh," Mike agreed quietly. "Only mine died."

"Mine lived." Jon was quiet for a minute. "When Jobi was sick, I was scared I'd get cancer too."

"Yeah, when my sister died, I knew anyone could die. I was scared, but I'm not any more."

"Me either. Let's go hit a few."

"Okay. I want to make majors this year."

252

"Me too."

Children know about life going on.

Next to Jonathan would sit Heidi, my lovely teenage daughter. I could visualize her brooding blue eyes and the graceful movements of her tall figure. She would be sixteen soon, but had yet to discover her self-worth. She was too busy with her anger toward all of us; toward Jobi for the same old reasons, toward Jon for his closeness to David, toward me for being unequal to the task of filling her needs. Yet I was sure of the keen intelligence behind that troubled forehead; the capacity for love masked by her often cold expression.

Heidi liked us to think she didn't love her sister, but she had inadvertently revealed her true feelings one day. A boy had chased Jobi with a metal stick. Jobi was on her bicycle, which she rode expertly, but her fear of the stick in the boy's hand had caused her to take her eyes from the street and look back at her pursuer. Her bike collided with that of another child who was coming down the street. The two children went down in the gravelly road, both bikes falling on top of Jobi. Her face, back, arms, and leg were badly cut. Blood and dirt covered her. I heard the children screaming and ran out into the street. On that early summer evening, a party was going on. Heidi and her friends were dancing on the patio in back of the house. When she heard the commotion, Heidi came running around the house. She looked at Jobi still lying in the street and listened to the hysterically related story of the accident. Heidi's face became enraged. Tears of mixed pity and anger filled her eyes.

"I'm going to find the kid who did this to her and kill him," she said harshly. It was all I could do to stop her from leaving her friends and going on her mission of revenge. But at least I knew Heidi's secret—she really did care about her sister.

Heidi still had a long way to go toward learning to express and accept love, but progress had been made. She let me touch her now, and sometimes even touched me in return. There was promise in this volcanic child of mine.

I had reached the setting at the head of the table. I paused and touched the back of the chair where someone very special would sit tonight. It would not be David who celebrated Jobi's triumph with us. David had left me two years before. The leaving was not unexpected; the signs were present almost immediately after Jobi seemed out of danger. At first I had been devastated, thinking perhaps Lois had been right so long ago. Perhaps the terrible illness of a child had the power to destroy the marriage of the parents. But placing the blame for a bad relationship on the frail shoulders of a little girl was neither fair nor accurate. Our marriage had been tenuous long before Jobi's surgery. Our child's disease had only delayed the inevitable divorce, not caused it. The effect of the ordeal David suffered was reflected only, perhaps, in the woman he chose to replace me. She was lovely, young, athletic, and served him no reminder of illness or despair.

When David had left behind his bad memories, he had also relinquished his place in the celebration. Sitting beside me that night would be my husband of only six weeks, Joel Waller.

I met Joel at a party. My bachelor uncle, Frank, had persuaded me to come to the singles party even though I tried to resist. I looked at all the separated and divorced people trying to appear as though they were having fun, and I nearly ran from the room. I hid in a corner, hoping no one would talk to me. Maybe Frank would want to leave early.

Two cowboy-booted toes appeared in the spot on the floor at which I had been staring most of the evening. I looked up to see a darkly bearded face with smiling blue eyes and very white teeth.

"I think we should be dancing," the man said in a deep resonant voice.

Next Joel thought we should be having coffee together,

then he thought we should be dating every night, and finally, he thought we should be married. I agreed in every instance. It wasn't easy for Joel, marrying me and my package. Heidi resented his intrusion into our lives, and Jon, while amicable enough, worshipped his father too much to allow any real relationship between himself and his stepfather. But Jobi had room for everyone, and she and Joel bestowed unbridled affection on each other.

On one of the plates at the table sat a tiny package. It was wrapped in yellow paper and tied with a red ribbon . . . a gift to Jobi from my mother and father. I knew that inside the box was a delicate gold ring with one small but shining diamond—Jobi's birthstone. When Jobi saw the ring, her eyes would light, the golden flecks in the circles of blue becoming more pronounced. A dimple would appear as her smile spread, and her cheeks would flush pinkly. I knew she would rise from her chair and throw her arms around her grandparents, first one and then the other, kissing and thanking like champagne bubbles bursting. I knew all of these things would happen because she was Jobi.

Jobi. She was lightning and she was clouds. She could touch your cheek with fingertips like flower petals, and she could stand with fists clenched in fierce defiance if her abilities were challenged.

A foolish doctor had reminded her that she was an above-knee amputee and told her she could never roller-skate. Her next birthday party was a roller-skating party and she skated . . . with help at first, then alone and triumphant.

Al Pike, prosthetist at the Winkley Company, wanted Jobi to learn to ski. Dr. McMillan feared she would injure her only leg and advised against skiing. I left the decision to Jobi. Jobi's skiing adventures were featured in a local newspaper, and she was interviewed on a television show called "The Ski Scene."

Amputees can't dance. But Jobi dances. When I watched her dance across the stage in a United Synagogue Youth production of "Mame," wearing an artistically shaped foam prosthesis, I cried. Jobi didn't cry—she smiled radiantly and flirted a little with the boy next to her on stage.

After Jobi's surgery, I had worried about her future sensuality. I needn't have worried. She's curvy and provocative, and many young men are attracted to her. Of course, some are not. One day a boy on whom she had a crush took her to a party. Everything was fine until Jobi sat on the boy's lap. He recoiled from the touch of her prosthesis and never came near her again. She was heartbroken until the following week, when another boy took her to a dance and looked at her with shining eyes.

I have been criticized for the way I raised my amputee daughter. I have been accused of neglecting to tell her she was handicapped. I am guilty. I never told her. I never will.

Someone asked me once, "What saved Jobi?" Was it David's perseverance . . . was it Dr. Wilbur's medicine . . . was it my refusal to let her go . . . was it the family's love . . . was it Jobi's will to live? I'm not sure. It was all those things and more.

Recently Dr. Wilbur told me that Adriamycin and methotrexate are being used with great effectiveness on children with bone cancer, yet there are major medical centers in this country where doctors don't use chemotherapy because they don't think it will help. He explained a new method of treating teenagers who contract osteogenic sarcoma. The tumor and part of the bone are removed and a metal pipe is used to replace the missing bone section. The results have been more than promising, yet most doctors regard the procedure as too risky and too controversial . . . they amputate limbs instead.

No, I don't know what saved Jobi, but I know it wasn't a decision to take no action. I know it wasn't an attitude of fear toward risk and controversy. And it certainly wasn't a negative approach to disease. My blood runs cold when I hear of doctors who tell their patients that there is no hope for them, and I'm filled with anger when I see well-meaning volunteers come to talk to cancer victims about death and dying. I feel infinite pity for people who give up before they even fight.

This book is an affirmation of life and the pursuit of living it. The night of the celebration of Jobi's life, our family sat in a circle around the table. We spoke of the hope required to save a life and the strength needed for living it.

January 18, 1980

Dear Jo Anna,

Well, anyway, hello. It's funny to me how people get to know each other so well, spending great amounts of crucial time in their lives together, then get separated and never see or hear from each other . . . not even knowing who goes where, who has done what or who has lived.

I was thinking about the things that have happened to me because my mom is writing a book about me. Guess what? You're in it. That's why I was thinking about you.

Hmmm, I don't know where to start. I know one thing— no matter how hard things are, I feel extremely lucky. I made it. Here I am fifteen years old (sixteen in April— yeah, driving!), and I *really am here.* I'm kind of scared also. I *think* I know where I'm going, I only hope I can get there.

I really would like to grow up and be a surgeon (first I must grow up, not too fast, as my parents insist on reminding me). I'm not quite sure why I picked surgeon, but I've always known that's what I want to be. It's kind of stuck inside me and it will never go away, not until I reach my goal.

Let me tell you about myself right now. I'm a tenth grader at Armstrong Senior High School. I guess it's a pretty good school. I'm taking American Literature, American history, Algebra II, Modern Biology, French (fifth year already), and gym. My teachers are pretty OK, except for my history teacher, Mr. Florman. He's more than OK; he's one of the best teachers in the school.

School does have a few major-turned-minor problems for me. There are four floors to our school and *lots* of staircases. We shall overcome! The other biggie is that my last class ends at the time school lets out, and it's on the top floor. My locker is completely on the other side of the building, and my bus is all the way across the parking lot and leaves first. Problem solved; my jacket goes to math with me so I don't have to go back to my locker.

There are a few irritating things in my school—the people who treat me differently. God, I hate being different. Don't get me wrong—when I walk into a room and people turn around because they think I'm gorgeous (this is not a common occurrence, only a fantasy), that kind of attention I *love*. And when people gather around me because I'm being witty, charming, and bubbly (more fantasy), that kind of attention I like. But I'll be damned if I'm gonna ever again get attention by sitting in a wheelchair at Disneyland, even if it *is* just because my leg hurts so much. Never again will I go to school without my leg on, or be embarrassed by swimming in public, because I don't *have* to be different.

Last year a new leg became available to me. It has a foam cover and looks and feels 72% real, in comparison to the old one at 24%. My mom agreed that I should have it, but my dad didn't. It was an out-and-out battle, but now I'm 48% less different.

I have a difficulty though; I don't tell most people the truth about myself anymore. If a casual acquaintance asks me why I limp, I don't like to embarrass them or me, so I make something up; something athletic—guys like that better. I say I had a tennis or skiing accident. My mom agrees. When someone asks her why she limps she tells them it's an old football injury. But my dad thinks it's terrible and that I should see a psychiatrist. I think differently.

Nobody wants another heartache, and some people scare off easily. Let them know me mentally before physically—then they can make an honest decision whether to be my friend. Some do decide no, unfortunately. Mostly guys. I've had some difficulty accepting it, but in the same position, I don't know how I'd react, so I let it ride. Sometimes I win, sometimes I lose.

The real people never stop caring. My friends all have been great. It must have been hard sometimes. I was pretty temperamental; still am, I guess. Too much "special treatment"? I get along.

It's kinda hard telling people about me—where do you start? Never scare them away, make them care more; take you for what you are—right? This isn't so easy.

This summer I'm supposed to go to USY camp. God, I haven't been to camp in a long time. I'm really scared. Running around in public in shorts? Swimming? I am so self-conscious lately. I don't even ski anymore because I don't like to go out without my leg on. Pretty shabby, huh? Maybe not. Maybe I'm just growing up. I'm melting in, being recognized. Next time I'm in the papers, it's gonna be for modeling or because I discover the cure for cancer or something. Me—not the little blond girl who's an amputee.

I don't know where you live, Jo Anna, so I'm gonna send this letter in care of Dr. Wilbur and hope he can get it to you. Please write back and tell me about yourself.

I was just reading over the last pages of my mother's book. How strange—it's my life story. But how could it be? I'm only fifteen, and I have my whole life in front of me. Thank God.

Your friend,

Jobi Halper